GETTING
BUILT

GETTING BUILT

Dr. Lynne Pirie
with Bill Reynolds

WARNER BOOKS

A Warner Communications Company

The author gratefully acknowledges the following publishers for granting permission to reproduce illustrations:
B. G. King and M. J. Showers, *Human Anatomy and Physiology,* 6th Ed., Philadelphia: W. B. Saunders Co., 1969.
James E. Crouch, *Essential Human Anatomy,* Philadelphia: Lea & Febiger, 1982.

Warner Books, Inc., 666 Fifth Avenue, New York, NY 10103

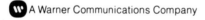 A Warner Communications Company

Printed in the United States of America

First printing: April 1984

10 9 8 7 6 5 4

Designed by Giorgetta Bell McRee

LIBRARY OF CONGRESS CATALOGING IN PUBLICATION DATA

Pirie, Lynne.
  Getting built.

  Bibliography: p. 205
  1. Bodybuilding for women. 2. Exercise for women.
I. Title.
GV546.6.W64P57   1984   646.7'5   83-26002
ISBN 0-446-38289-2 (U.S.A.) (pbk.)
      0-446-38290-6 (Canada) (pbk.)

To my loving and supportive husband,
John Kent Schmelzer

Special thanks to:

Mr. Jerry Doyle—my coach, whose dedicated efforts can never be repaid. Without you my success would never have occurred.

Ms. Cindy Van Baalen—who typed the original manuscript. A true friend whose efforts are sincerely appreciated.

Ms. Terry Doyle—Jerry's daughter and right arm. Thank you for your never-ending support and encouragement.

Ms. Kathy Simmons—Managing Editor, Warner Books, New York. You had faith in me to write this book and provided immense support and guidance. Without your superb expertise this book would not have been written.

CONTENTS

GETTING BUILT

INTRODUCTION

This book is dedicated to women of all ages, fitness levels, and body types who want to dramatically improve their figures, posture, health, strength, and body image and do so as quickly as possible. It is devised to serve both the athlete involved in competitive bodybuilding and the previously untrained individual.

I've written from the heart as much as from the head. Why? Because I *love* bodybuilding. There is no other activity like it. I know. My premedical student years were spent in undergraduate- and graduate-level programs in physical education, kinesiology, and exercise physiology. I competed in a number of varsity sports and participated in a vast array of other forms of exercise. Nothing else comes close. *Nothing.*

I have known hundreds of women from a variety of sports backgrounds (including some whose primary exercise was skipping gym class) who have been absolutely amazed at the effect that weight training has on figure development. They have been delighted at the positive health benefits that accompany bodybuilding. It feels good! You're lithe, vibrant, in control, unbeatable. You develop a heightened body awareness that serves as a potent motivational force, driving you through each workout in pursuit of physical excellence. Once you've begun to realize the benefits, you're hooked. There is no substitute.

I started bodybuilding at age eighteen, during my sophomore year in college. As a member of the varsity women's basketball team, I suddenly became aware of a glaring lack of upper body strength. So did my coach. My legs were beginning to look a little "loose" in the thighs, too, even though I wasn't what you'd call fat. I was already running two to three miles a day!

My coach, Miss Dresser, marched me into the college's weight room and demonstrated four or five exercises that would increase my upper body strength. Then she walked out, leaving me the only female there. The football players and wrestlers were mildly amused. Not me. No strength, no baskets...and no starting position on the team. So three days a week I went to the weight room and did my workout. It took about fifteen minutes. And I found I was getting stronger. Shots from ten and fifteen feet out were not only making it to the basket, they often went through. Swish! And my rebound skills were improving at the same time.

1

As I continued weight training, I watched some of the men and picked up a few new exercises for other body parts—stomach muscles, legs, and calves. Soon my workouts were lasting a half hour. I felt great. My tummy was getting flatter; my legs were rapidly improving—no more ripples. Even my bust line was changing. There was a new fullness in my chest that was quite flattering—even a little hint of cleavage. All this after a mere two months. Amazing! This was for me. A Mark Eden invention that had been purchased some time before and proved ineffective was unceremoniously tossed out.

The men in the weight room noticed the difference, too. Several commented that they would like to see their girlfriends begin to use weights. Talk about positive reinforcement! And the results came so much more quickly than I had expected. Even my running was improving. Some of my female classmates became interested.

When the spring term ended and it was time to go home for the summer, the first thing I did was find a job. The next was to find a gym. At that time, less than fifteen years ago, it was a miracle in a small town of 50,000 to find a gym where women were encouraged to use weights. I was fortunate to find a beautiful, immaculate gym, fully equipped with all the weights I would ever need. It was owned by Jim and Julia Pappas, a husband and wife team who had been involved with men's bodybuilding since that sport's inception.

Julia took me under her wing, introducing me to a basic program that included one or two exercises for each major muscle group. Each workout was the same, involving the entire body. Soon my best friend joined me. We pushed each other and steadily increased our work load. We were looking better and better, toned and tanned. What a summer! We've been lifting weights ever since. Seeing the potential for figure development through weight training, my new axiom was "Behind every worthwhile curve is a muscle." I adhere to that principle more today than ever.

When you're a young, fresh teenager—up to fourteen or fifteen—youth is on your side. Muscle tone, size, and strength are probably the best they will ever be without some kind of strenuous exercise routine. However, as time marches on, the effects of gravity, our relatively sedentary lifestyle, and America's favorite fast foods begin to make their impression (or depressions)—sagging and flattened buttocks and breasts, protruding abdomens, cellulite-laden thighs complete with "saddlebags."

The problems seem to develop overnight. Time to diet and exercise, you tell yourself. But, as you probably already know, the amount of dieting necessary to alleviate flabby thighs generally leaves you fatigued, weak, and irritable. Your face begins to look "too thin," as your friends will be sure to tell you. Your bra looks two sizes too big, and someone will probably mention that, too. This wasn't quite the look you had in mind. You ask yourself, Why do I have to emaciate my upper body in order to get my thighs and hips reduced to desirable proportions? The answer is simple: You don't have to. What you really need to do is establish a better balance between upper and lower body development. Most women don't have a sufficient amount of upper body muscle, and that lack is accentuated when following conventional dieting routines.

Traditionally delicate creatures, we women have never been encouraged to develop our musculature, particularly in our chest, back, arms, and shoulders. If the cap on a bottle of ketchup was "too tight," the thing to do was blink helplessly while some man accomplished the necessary feat of strength for us. Girls weren't supposed to have muscles. And then don't forget the myth that girls/women who played sports that were physically demanding somehow lost their femininity.

Even for most athletic women, upper body strength and muscular development were not required for success. And so it was that at age fourteen or fifteen the vast majority peaked physically in terms of muscularity. After that, gradual deterioration as the old "what you don't use you lose" adage proved itself true.

Most women don't notice the loss in upper body musculature, since fat continues to increase, with no appreciable loss of body size evident. However, when a diet strips away this layer of fat, all that is left are some thin, poorly shaped muscles and bone—not very attractive. What you really wanted was a full, healthy, toned look, bursting with sensual vitality. But achieving this desired appearance requires an optimal amount of well-shaped, well-placed muscle as well as sensible dietary practices.

I have always admired the bodies of top gymnasts and dancers. But they train five to eight hours a day. Few of us have more than sixty to ninety minutes to invest daily in the pursuit of exercise. This is where the magic of bodybuilding comes in. A specifically designed program can yield outstanding results in terms of selective muscle development. Bodybuilding is the most efficient and effective method of reshaping and contouring the human physique to ideal proportions. In fact, it is the *only* way, and it is very healthy.

Since seeing is believing, here's a picture of me when I was seventeen years old. I'm the one at the top left-hand side of the pyramid. Compare this to a recent picture taken fifteen years later. Judge for yourself. Who has the better body, the seventeen-year-old or the thirty-two-year-old? The remarkable thing is that approximately 60 percent of the improvement was achieved in the year prior to this writing, when I markedly altered

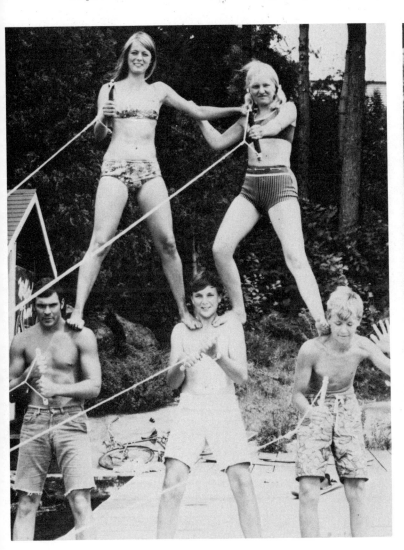 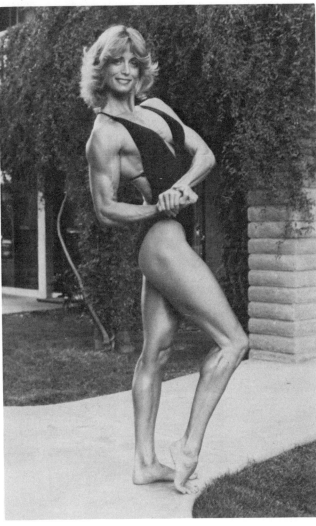

Who has the better body, the seventeen-year-old or the thirty-two-year-old?

my training program. That was at the prompting of my present coach, Jerry Doyle, of Phoenix, Arizona. Under his expert tutelage the gains I've made have been phenomenal. To illustrate the difference he's made, compare the next two pictures—before Doyle and after Doyle.

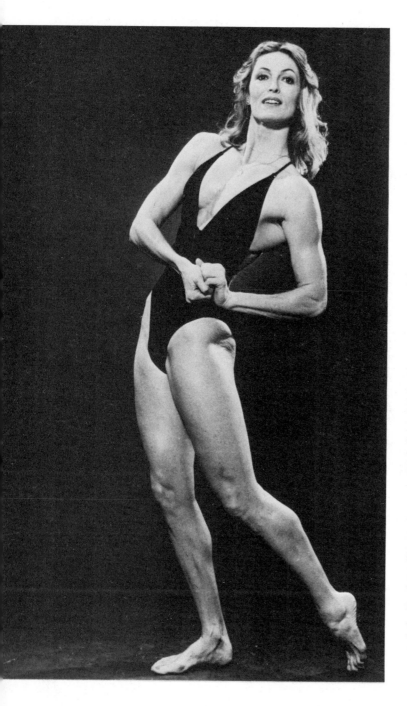
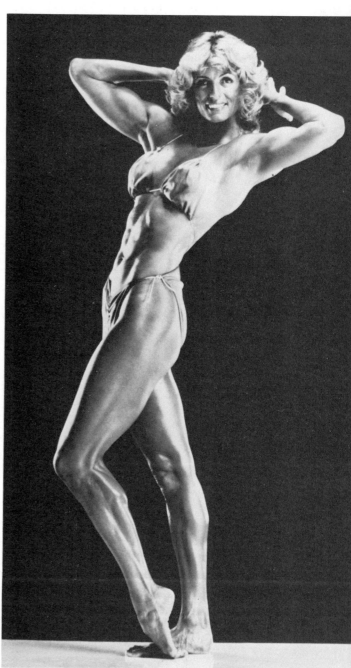

Before Doyle and after Doyle.

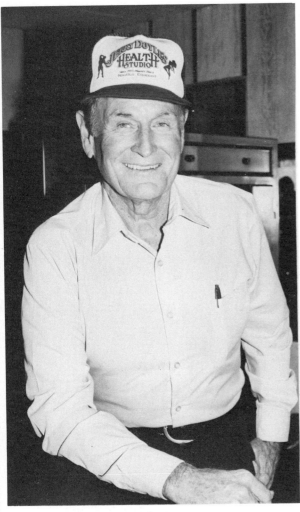

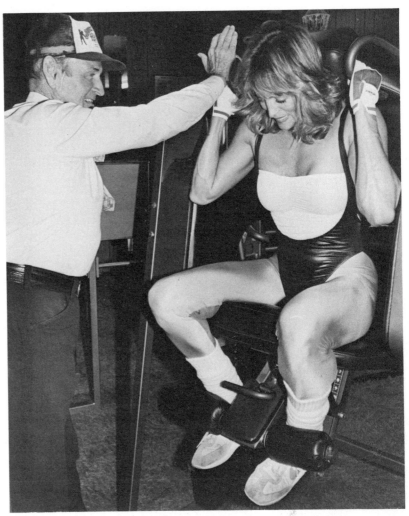

My coach, Jerry Doyle.

Jerry applies additional resistance on high-intensity Nautilus crunches.

The Pirie-Doyle training methods are described in complete, comprehensive detail in this book. Regardless of your present body type (fat or thin) or previous activity patterns (sedentary or national class athlete), the intelligent use of the bodybuilding techniques presented here will prove the fastest, surest means of totally remodeling your body to achieve optimum tone, size, and proportions.

The woman of the eighties is strong, healthy, capable—a tigress who rules her own world. The attitudes of the fifties, which kept her a fatty pair of breasts and hips, or those of the sixties, which promoted a spindly twig silhouette, have been defeated. Women are now able to pursue freely the paths that lead to the exultant achievement of optimum potential—spiritual, mental, and physical. A strong, healthy, well-proportioned, athletic-looking body is finally "in." Unlike its predecessors, it is the product of an aggressively healthy lifestyle that feels good!

You can be confident that this approach to fitness is not just a passing fad. We women are no longer afraid to be naturally beautiful. In fact we're training like fighters to be so.

This book will give you a firm foundation of basic knowledge for achievement of your physical potential through bodybuilding. It's organized to provide you an understanding of your body's structure and needs as well as to give you a complete set of training routines to build with.

5

The human body is a wonder. I say that both as a bodybuilder and as an orthopedic surgeon. With each day I find myself more than ever convinced of the genius and power of God, who has given us the amazing gift of the human body. It is a gift too many of us take for granted. Any machine as neglected and abused as the average person's body is would have ceased functioning long ago. Fortunately, our body's capacity to recover and repair itself repeatedly saves us from our own unwitting self-destruction. Isn't it time for you to show some appreciation for this blessing by taking the initiative to promote your body's optimal functioning? The best medicine is still prevention, and bodybuilding is great medicine, without bitter taste or adverse side effects. The prescription is here for you. Enjoy!

GETTING TO KNOW YOUR BODY | 1

In order to understand what bodybuilding can do for you, you first have to understand some basic points about your body and how it works. In particular, you have to know something about your natural line of build and about your own muscle structure. While bodybuilding provides a means for remarkable change through muscle development, it's not a form of magic. You can only work with what you have; you can't create something out of nothing.

YOUR BODY TYPE

Take a look at yourself in the mirror. What do you see your basic build to be? Are you a round, plump individual and have been that way all your life? Are you essentially a muscular person by heredity? Or are you a thin person with long, thin arms and legs?

These three general descriptions correlate to three different qualities of physique: *endomorphy*, which refers to the relative amount of fat you have; *mesomorphy*, which refers to the amount of muscle you have; and *ectomorphy*, which is an expression of thinness of body parts.

Very few people can be termed either all endomorph, all mesomorph, or all ectomorph, the body types in which the particular indicated characteristic clearly predominates. You are probably best described in terms of a combination of two or more of these characteristics. Most people's physiques fall into a pattern of relative predominance in one area, with secondary characteristics evident from another area. Some physiologists use a numerical coding to define individual body types, assigning a value to the evident degree of endomorphy, mesomorphy, and ectomorphy in each case. Say the scale runs from 1 to 7, with 7 indicating maximum evidence of the particular body trait. Your rating might be 2-5-2—fairly low in body fat, relatively muscular, and not evidencing a particular thinness in your build. (The number sequence refers to endomorphy, mesomorphy, and ectomorphy in that sequence.)

Determining actual numerical values for each aspect of your physique would require an assessment using photographs and actual measurements, with reference to scientifically determined base types. That is likely to be beyond you. But you can assess your own build roughly by evaluating your reflection in a mirror.

Do you have long thin limbs or short limbs? That will determine if you are mainly ectomorphic or not. Now, we're not asking if you're tall or short; it's a question of proportion. The ectomorphy rating is based primarily on height-to-weight ratios (height divided by the cube root of weight). Of course, ectomorphy is most obvious with tall people who have a very linear appearance, but a very thin short person is also properly characterized as an ectomorph.

Do you have a more obvious thickness in your bone structure, with a heavier musculature and not too much body fat? Then you are more of a mesomorph. As the body fat becomes more pronounced, you move over to being considered an endomorph.

Probably you'll see yourself as combining two qualities. If you are a chubby person with a strong secondary muscular component, you're a mesomorphic endomorph. If you're fairly muscular but with a noticeable secondary chubbiness, then you're an endomorphic mesomorph.

The balanced mesomorph—strong in muscularity and neither noticeably fat or thin to any degree—will have a very appealing athletic appearance. The ectomorphic mesomorph, a muscular person but with longer limbs than the balanced mesomorph, also presents a very appealing type of physique. The mesomorphic ectomorph is probably the most appealing of all. This person has long lean arms, legs, and torso and yet has nice muscular development. The difference between this body type and the ectomorphic mesomorph is that the latter will be somewhat more muscular than the former.

How much can you change your basic physique? Well, there's some argument about that. What is certain is that you can change the balance to a considerable degree in some areas.

Certainly you can change the amount of fat that you have underneath your skin. While the evidence indicates that fat cells are not destroyed through weight loss, they do change in size—that is, grow larger or smaller. There is an appetite control mechanism in the body that is sensitive to the size of fat cells and that has a feeling for how large your fat cells should be, based upon what you have kept them at for any substantial length of time. That is why it can be very hard to keep yourself down to a level of leanness after being on a diet. Your body's tendency is to return to what has come to be its "normal" condition. If your fat cells have been enlarged for a long time, the body perceives that as normal and through biochemical means prompts you to eat enough to regain that "normal" size. However, if you can hold weight down for a prolonged period of time, gradually your body comes to accept the lower fat levels as normal.

There is not much you can do about your bone structure once you stop growing. However, with weight training, bone structure will be preserved and possibly somewhat enhanced in response to the activity demands placed on it. Obviously the length of limbs cannot be changed short of surgery. However, their relative thinness can be changed by changing the amount of fat or muscle on them.

Bodybuilding, of course, particularly emphasizes the potential for change in musculature. Your degree of mesomorphy can be altered through applied effort. Much as with the degree of endomorphy, the level of change must be maintained through a constant use of the involved muscle at the increased rate, or your body will revert back to its previously "normal" state.

While bodybuilding is primarily associated with a buildup of muscle mass, as a
8   bodybuilder you will actually be concerned with both aspects of build subject to your con-

trol, limiting endomorphy and achieving greater mesomorphy. We'll emphasize muscle development in the pages that follow, but we'll also look at dietary factors you must attend to if you hope to achieve your best physical potential. You can't trade in your body for a wholly new one, but you can do a major reconstruction job on the body you have.

HOW YOUR MUSCLES WORK

The dominant theme in this book is muscle development, specifically the development of skeletal muscle. (Your body also contains involuntary smooth muscles in the gut and the specialized cardiac muscle that makes up the heart. While the health of these muscles is affected by your general state of health and physical condition, you cannot control them directly, as you can the voluntary skeletal muscles.)

The clearly apparent role of skeletal muscle is to produce movement at a joint. As a rule, a muscle can only act on the joint(s) that it crosses. It works primarily by contracting, shortening to increase tension across the joint, thereby pulling the body parts that meet at the joint closer together. For example, flexing your biceps muscle results in a contraction that pulls the forearm up toward the upper arm.

Of course, a muscle also has to work to manage tension at a point where the fibers themselves must expand. For example, if you perform a push-up, you will notice that your arm and elbow straighten as you reach the top of the movement. That is largely through the contracting power of the triceps muscle. The force of its contraction is what extends the elbow. When you lower yourself in the downward position of the movement cycle, the triceps has to lengthen in order to allow bending at the elbow. It cannot simply relax, or you would fall on your face. A certain tension has to be maintained, allowing a gradual giving way to the force of gravity. This kind of tension is known as an eccentric contraction. The muscle gives in to gravity but acts to manage the response.

Bodybuilders often perform exercises in which there is tension in a muscle but the muscle fibers are lengthening rather than contracting. Say you are doing a machine curl. When you pull the bar up toward you, the muscle is contracting. But then if you exert as much force as you can to keep the bar up while a training partner pulls down on it to the extent that she overcomes your force, the muscle necessarily lengthens, even though it seeks to maintain contraction. This type of stimulus, where the muscle is forced to lengthen while seeking to maintain contraction, is termed "negative" force in bodybuilding. It places a maximum demand on the muscle involved, stimulating further development as the muscle seeks to respond to the overload by compensating growth. Many bodybuilders rely on negative force exercises to stimulate muscles to maximum growth.

There are times when a muscle tries to contract to accomplish movement but cannot. That results in an isometric contraction. For example, if I try to pick a weight up off the floor but can't move it, I'm performing an isometric action. The muscles are tensing with a maximum effort at contraction, but they aren't actually shortening or lengthening. (An actual shortening or lengthening response is termed an isotonic action.) Because an isometric contraction involves maximum effort to overcome resistance, isometric exercises can be valuable for inducing muscle growth. As an example, some athletes have a weak spot in the initiation of movement when it comes to performing curls or bench presses—they can't get the barbell to move that first inch. So they practice pushing as hard as they can against a bar that is too heavy for them to move in order to build strength at this point.

Muscles also function to provide joint stability. That is, they tense in order to hold a joint in a fixed position. When you are working with weights, the muscles that do the work of moving the barbell will be the only ones in motion. That does not mean they are the only ones working. Other muscles are maintaining you in a sufficiently rigid stance so that you hold your balance in whatever position you've assumed for the exercise.

Of course, muscles work together, often in complementary fashion. The muscle that is involved in producing a given movement is called the "prime mover." The muscle that would produce the opposite movement is called the "opponent" or "antagonist." A muscle that helps a given action to be performed but is not the prime mover is called a "synergist."

The end of any muscle attached to the bone that does not move when the muscle is contracted is termed its "origin." The end attached to the bone that moves is its "insertion." Using the biceps as an example again, the origin is in the upper arm–shoulder area;

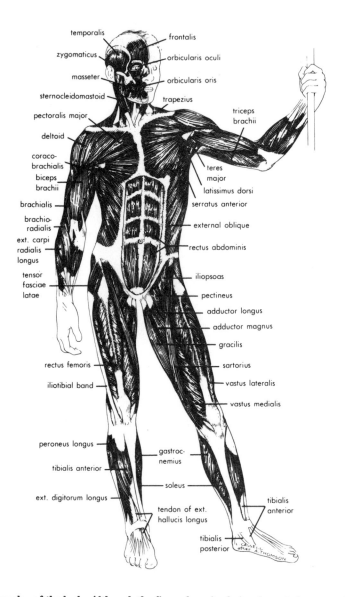

Anterior view of muscles of the body. Although the figure here is obviously male in proportion, the body muscles are all the same except for a few, not shown here, in the genital area. (From King, B. G., and Showers, M. J., *Human Anatomy and Physiology*, 6th edition, Philadelphia: W. B. Saunders, 1969. Reproduced with permission.)

Posterior view of the muscles of the body. (From King, B. G., and Showers, M. J., *Human Anatomy and Physiology,* 6th edition, Philadelphia: W. B. Saunders, 1969. Reproduced with permission.)

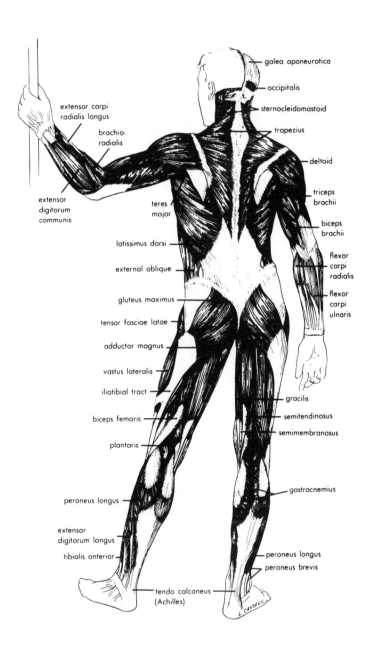

the insertion is on the radius of the forearm. When you contract your biceps, you raise the forearm while the upper arm–shoulder remains relatively fixed in position. In some cases, depending on the movement, the point of origin and point of insertion may be reversed. If you are doing sit-ups, your upper body moves while the legs remain relatively fixed. When you are doing leg raises, you use some of the same muscles, but now the legs move while the upper body remains relatively fixed.

Muscles attach to bones by means of tendons, wide fibrous tissue sheaths called aponeuroses, or by fleshy attachments directly to the bone itself. Although the muscles that they anchor are capable of contraction, tendons and aponeuroses are not.

11

Other important structures in relation to muscles are bursae and synovial sheaths. The bursae are fluid-filled sacs that lie between tendons and bones or between muscle groups themselves to ease the sliding of one over the other. Synovial sheaths are a kind of tunnel through which a tendon runs to its connection with a bone. Their purpose is also to allow movement with a minimum of friction. Most people are unaware of the important role played by bursae and synovial sheaths until they suffer bursitis or tendinitis, conditions of inflammation of these structures that can be very painful.

THE MAJOR MUSCLES AND MUSCLE GROUPS

A bodybuilder has to be concerned with development of all the major muscle groups in the body. No one area can be ignored, or her appearance will turn out unbalanced. Many recreational bodybuilders—traditionally men—concentrate on developing their arms and chests while ignoring their backs and legs. Women are sometimes guilty of the same failure to balance development. I cannot stress too highly the importance of training all the muscle groups if you wish to attain the most desirable results.

Let's briefly run though the major muscles/muscle groups that you should pay attention to. I'll provide a capsule description of the origin, insertion, and action of each, as these points of information are important for selecting exercises that ensure a balanced development. Refer to the accompanying illustrations to sharpen your understanding of the details given here.

THE ARM

Deltoids

These are the muscles that give much of the roundness at the point on either side where the arm meets the shoulder. They have their origin at the upper extreme of the shoulder blade, where it meets the collarbone. On each side they are made up of three heads that

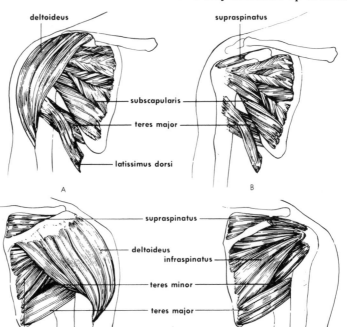

The deltoid and adjoining muscles in the shoulder area. *A*, viewed from the front. *B*, viewed from the back.

weave together to insert in progression on the bone of the upper arm. The main action of the deltoid is to raise the arm, but it requires the coordinated activity of several muscles to accomplish this. The deltoid plays its role once the motion has been initiated and can then raise the arm to shoulder level. Other muscles must take over to raise it higher. The deltoid also plays a role in flexing, extending, and rotating the arm.

The fibers that make up the posterior head are used relatively little in raising the arm, so these will not develop if exercise in a shoulder routine concentrate only on raising the arm overhead. The posterior fibers play more of a role in pulling the arm back to the side. Since gravity makes this easy as a rule, you won't get full development unless you specifically work the muscle against resistance.

Biceps

The biceps has two heads. The long head has its origin by the cavity of the shoulder blade in which the upper arm bone (the humerus) is inserted. The short head has its origin on an adjacent ridge of the shoulder blade. Both heads come together to form a muscle belly about one-third of the way down the arm and insert via a common tendon onto the bones of the forearm. With maximum development, the split between the two heads before they merge is readily apparent, and this is considered an asset in competitive bodybuilding. You will also see one muscle belly assume a slightly different contour where the two heads join, giving the appearance of a little hill sitting on top of a larger hill. This is also considered a competitive advantage.

Brachialis

This muscle lies beneath the biceps and attaches along the lower half of the humerus at the front. It inserts at the upper end of the ulna, one of the two bones in the forearm. Together with the biceps, it acts to flex the arm. You have to develop this muscle in order to display maximum biceps development.

Triceps

These are the muscles of the back of the upper arms. The triceps has three heads. Only the long head attaches to the shoulder blade. The other two heads originate from the back side of the humerus. The insertion is at the top of the bone comprising the elbow. The triceps muscles act to extend the arm and forearm. The long head also pulls the arm back when it's been raised away from the body.

The Forearm

The muscles here are basically used for extension and flexion. The extensors are located on the back and the flexors on the palm side of the forearm. We won't name them individually. Suffice it to say that they should not be neglected, as an arm will look very unbalanced with well-developed triceps and biceps and a thin, undeveloped forearm.

THE CHEST AREA

Intercostals

These are the muscles between each pair of ribs. They are arranged in two layers—the external intercostals and the internal intercostals—which are at right angles to each other. They raise the ribs to assist the diaphragm with forced respiration, particularly when inhaling. They are not much used by sedentary individuals, but with athletic activity that requires deep breathing or even forced breathing, they do come into play. They may become sore if an individual has not used them to any extent previously.

Pectoralis major

This fan-shaped muscle has its origin along the open line of the "fan" that spreads from the collarbone (claricle) along the breastbone (sternum) to the cartilage connecting the upper seven ribs to the breastbone. This muscle has two heads: the clavicular head and the sternal head. The former is the smaller and is often termed the "upper pecs"; the latter is much larger and makes up the bulk of the fan spread. The upper pecs are often not

13

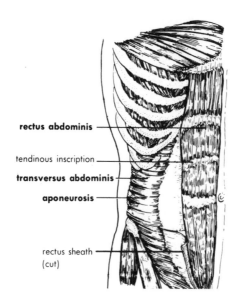

rectus abdominis

tendinous inscription

transversus abdominis

aponeurosis

rectus sheath
(cut)

The deep muscles of the abdominal wall.

The external and internal obliques in relation to other muscles in the abdomen and chest area.

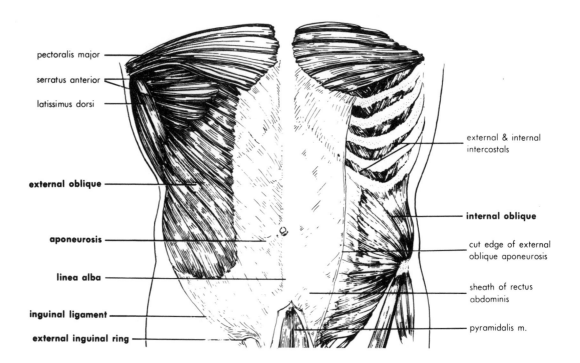

pectoralis major

serratus anterior

latissimus dorsi

external & internal
intercostals

external oblique

internal oblique

aponeurosis

cut edge of external
oblique aponeurosis

linea alba

sheath of rectus
abdominis

inguinal ligament

pyramidalis m.

external inguinal ring

given enough emphasis because of their lesser size, but their development is important for achieving fullness across the entire chest. The two heads cross and insert on the upper humerus. They come into play in all activities in which there is flexion or movement of the upper arm.

Known as "the fingers" in the upper chest, the serratus anterior originates from the outer surfaces of the eight upper ribs and inserts along the underside of the shoulder blade along the border closest to the spinal column. Although we do not exercise this muscle specifically, it is very important in stabilizing the shoulder girdle in all activities that involve upper body motion. As a result, it becomes developed quite easily, particularly through activities like bench pressing and dips.

Serratus anterior

THE ABDOMINAL AREA

This is a long powerful muscle that bodybuilders commonly refer to as the "abs." It is segmented, which is particularly evident in the "washboard stomach" characteristic of highly developed women bodybuilders. It arises from the fifth, sixth, and seventh ribs near where these join the breastbone and inserts on the pubic bone of the pelvis by means of a short tendon. This is the muscle that pulls your torso toward your lower body when doing sit-ups.

Rectus abdominus

This muscle has its origin from the side of the ribs and runs diagonally to insert on the sheath of fibrous tissue that surrounds the rectus abdominus. Its main role together with the internal oblique is to rotate the trunk. It also participates in flexing the torso.

External oblique

The internal oblique lies beneath the external oblique and runs at right angles to it. It is lower on the body, arising from the junction between the legs and the abdomen on either side, (the inguinal ligament), and it runs up toward the midline to fuse with the fibrous tissue that covers the rectus abdominus.

Internal oblique

The external and internal obliques and the fibrous tissue bands on which they insert form an anatomical girdle around the abdomen. It is the angle at which the two obliques slant toward each other that determines the hollow of the waist. Some individuals have a naturally smaller waist than others—the muscle fibers of their external and internal obliques run on a greater slant than those of persons with a thick waist.

It is important to realize that exercising your waist can thicken the muscle fibers here and destroy the hollow of your waist. Exercises that involve side-bending really do not benefit the obliques, as they do not exercise these muscles along their natural lines. Twisting exercises with little or no effort are the best for working the obliques. These give the muscles tone and prompt them to shorten, thereby drawing the waist in. With twisting motions, the external oblique on one side works in concert with the internal oblique on the other in order to rotate the torso.

This muscle runs across the abdominal wall from an origin along the side to insert in a line more or less along the midsection of the abdomen. It comes into play when you consciously pull your tummy in and is best exercised in your daily routine by doing this whenever you are sitting or standing. Keeping this muscle toned helps prevent a protruding stomach.

Transversus abdominis

THE BACK AREA   When a bodybuilder looks at her back, she concentrates on the muscles that provide width and on those that contribute to strength and development along the line from the shoulders to the hip areas. (While you might think to include the neck muscles among those to pay attention to, in general these do not need to be exercised separately for development. The most important thing for the neck muscles is to stretch them regularly to maintain a full range of movement that might otherwise be compromised by tension there.)

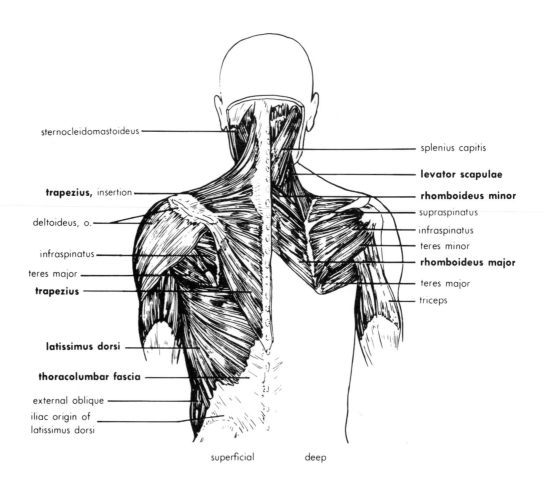

sternocleidomastoideus

splenius capitis

levator scapulae

trapezius, insertion

rhomboideus minor

supraspinatus

deltoideus, o.

infraspinatus

teres minor

infraspinatus

teres major

rhomboideus major

trapezius

teres major

triceps

latissimus dorsi

thoracolumbar fascia

external oblique

iliac origin of latissimus dorsi

superficial   deep

The muscles of the upper back.

Trapezius   The trapezius is a large, flat, triangular muscle that has its origin in a line along the spine from the back of the neck to the middle of the back itself. Its upper fibers insert on the end of the collarbone. The middle fibers run horizontally to insert on the spine of the shoulder blade, while the lower fibers run upward to insert right below those on the spine of the shoulder blade. Because of its wide origin, the muscle can work selectively in its various parts. It will therefore take a range of exercises to develop the entire muscle fully.

16   The upper fibers work to shrug the shoulders and pull the head back. The middle fibers pull the shoulders back (as with standing at attention) and also support the shoulder blade when the arm is raised above the head. The lower fibers assist in stabilizing the shoulder blade and pull it down as the arm is raised. The lower fibers are commonly very little developed in people who do not lift weights or perform any vigorous activity with their backs.

This muscle arises from connections with the first four cervical vertebrae (the upper spinal column) and inserts on the upper angle of the shoulder blade. It also acts to elevate or shrug the shoulders.

Levator scapulae

These are divided into the rhomboids minor and rhomboids major. They originate from the lower cervical vertebrae (still in the upper spinal column) and run obliquely to the side to insert where the shoulder blade borders on the spinal column. The rhomboids minor make up the smaller portion at the top; the rhomboids major are the larger portion directly beneath. They act to pull the shoulders back and to rotate the shoulder blade downward in connection with lowering the raised arm.

Rhomboids

These both originate at the lowest angle of the shoulder blade and the area immediately above and run to the side to insert on the humerus (the upper arm bone). The terres major inserts on the front of the humerus, the terres minor on the back. Together they act to rotate the arm and to pull it in toward the body.

Terres major and terres minor

This muscle actually lies underneath the shoulder blade, with its origin on the middle area and its insertion near the top of the humerus under the deltoid. It is important in rotating the shoulder and raising the arm.

Subscapularis

Another muscle that acts to rotate the shoulder and raise the arm, the supraspinatous has its origin in the area above the spine of the shoulder blade and also inserts near the top of the humerus.

Supraspinatous

The infraspinatous has its origin beneath the spine of the shoulder blade and inserts on the humerus at about the same spot as the supraspinatous. Its action is the same as the supraspinatous.

Infraspinatous

The terres minor, subscapularis, supraspinatous, and infraspinatous are collectively referred to as the *rotator cuff* because of their action together in rotating the shoulder. Injury to muscles in this joint area is common among athletes. It's ended the career of many a baseball pitcher and would seriously inhibit your working with weights. A tear in a muscle of the rotator cuff will make it impossible to raise a weight above shoulder level.

This is the muscle that gives the back its greatest width. (In Latin the name means "widest of the back.") It has the largest origin of all the muscles of the back, arising along the spinal column from a point just above the middle of the back to within a few inches of the tailbone. It progressively narrows as it runs upward and to the side toward the shoulder area, coming up from beneath to insert in a ribbonlike band about one inch wide on the front of the humerus. When it contracts, it pulls the shoulder back and downward; it also pulls the arm back toward the body, with some rotation. It has a secondary insertion on the lower angle of the shoulder blade near where the terres major originates. The "lats," as they are popularly termed among bodybuilders, are important in stabilizing the shoulder joints in bench pressing and push-ups.

Latissimus dorsi

17

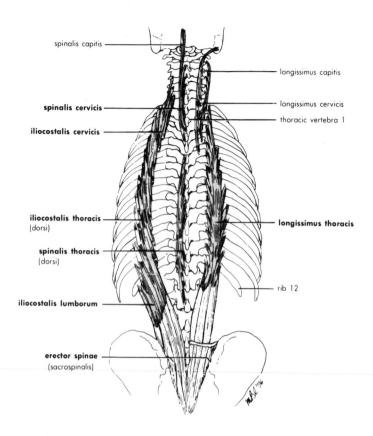

The erector spinae group of muscles. (The view is from the back.)

The erector spinae group

The erector spinae group is a combination of interacting muscles running on either side of the spinal column. They form two strong supporting pillars that are most evident in the lower back but actually extend the length of the back. They act to extend, side-bend, and rotate the lower back. In an unexercised person whose abdominals have poor tone or have been stretched by intraabdominal fat, the muscles of this group commonly become shortened and lose their flexibility. In conjunction with other muscles in the lower back weakening, this tends to increase the inward curve of the back, which places extra strain on the intervertebral discs in that area. This often results in the pain and muscle spasms characteristic of the all too common "low back syndrome."

THE HIP AREA

These are three in number: the gluteus maximus, gluteus medius, and gluteus minimus. (*Gluteus* is Latin for *rump*.)

The gluteal muscles

The gluteus maximus is one of the largest muscles in the body. It is placed entirely behind the hip joint. Its origin is on a broad line running from the iliac crest of the hipbone and curving down and inward to the tailbone. It inserts onto the upper shaft of the thighbone (femur), slightly in front of the outward protrusion known as the greater trochanter. (This is the protrusion you can feel on either side where the hip and thigh meet.) The gluteus maximus extends and rotates the thigh, but it is exerted with force only when power is demanded for activities like sprinting, squatting, or climbing stairs. It does not get much play when you are walking on a level surface.

The gluteus medius arises from the hipbone beneath the origin of the gluteus maximus and inserts on the top of the thighbone slightly on top of and in front of the greater trochanter. Its main action is to raise the leg out to the side and to help keep the hips level

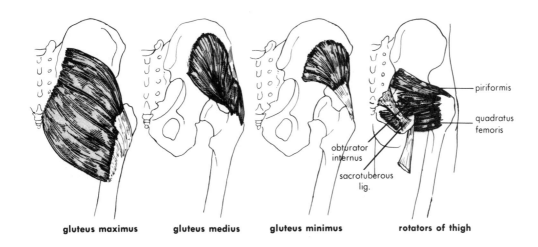

The gluteal muscles and lateral outward rotators.

when you transfer weight from one leg to another. You particularly work it with side leg raises.

The gluteus minimus originates from a somewhat more forward position on the iliac crest of the hipbone and inserts somewhat in front of the gluteus medius on the greater trochanter of the thighbone. Its actions are similar to those of the gluteus medius.

These are six small muscles with their origin beneath the gluteus maximus and inserting either onto the back of the thighbone proper near the top or onto the greater trochanter of the thighbone. They are important in extending the thigh and in outwardly rotating the hip joint. There is a very large nerve that passes in between these muscles that often becomes irritated in people who have lower back problems. *Lateral outward rotators*

The sartorius, which runs diagonally from its origin on the crest of the hipbone at the front of the hip to insert on the tibia of the lower leg near the inside of the knee, is the longest muscle in the body. It assists in flexing and rotating the thigh and leg. Although it is not a powerful muscle, it becomes very prominent in bodybuilders (particularly males) who have trained for competition. *THE THIGH*

Sartorius

This is actually a group of four muscles that run down the front of the thigh to insert on the kneecap. They all work to extend the leg. *Quadriceps femoris*

The rectus femoris originates on a ridge on the front of the hipbone. The tendon by which the muscle inserts on the kneecap actually wraps around the kneecap at the same time to anchor on the prominence of the knee formed by the top of the large bone of the lower leg (the tibia). This muscle also acts to flex the thigh.

The other three muscles are collectively known as the vasti. The vastus intermedius is located immediately beneath the rectus femoris. It has its origin on the shaft of the thighbone. The vastus lateralis, running along the outside of the thigh, originates on the greater trochanter of the thighbone. The vastus medialis originates on the upper inside of the thighbone. It attaches to the kneecap via the same tendon, and is very important in keep-

19

ing the kneecap properly centered. In many women, who have a greater angle from the hip to the knee than men do because of the greater width of the female pelvis, the vastus medialis may not be developed enough to keep the kneecap from dislocating with strenuous activity, and this can lead to painful difficulty when running or engaging in further activity. This dislocation can be complicated by erosion of the cartilage beneath the kneecap. Strengthening this muscle may help to correct the problem.

The adductors These are the muscles on the inside of the thigh that act to keep the knees pulled together. They all arise from the lower section of the pelvis known as the pubic ramis and insert at various inside positions along the shaft of the thighbone. They work to flex the thigh and in some cases to rotate it, as well as to pull the leg in. When these muscles are not developed, you often see a large space between the thighs, giving the appearance of being knock-kneed.

The hamstring muscles These are three muscles in the back of the thigh that work together to flex the knee, rotate the leg, and extend the hips. They originate from the bony prominence of the pelvis that you feel when you sit down. (It's often referred to as the "sit bone.")

The biceps femoris, located toward the outside of the thigh, has two heads. The long head has its origin along the "sit bone"; the short head arises along the middle of the thighbone. Together they insert on the upper portions of the tibia and fibula, the two bones of the lower leg. There is a wide variation from one individual to the next in the relationship between the two heads of the biceps femoris, much as with the biceps of the arm. In a well-developed athlete you can see the separation between the two heads, although that will be more apparent in some than in others.

The semimembranosus and semitendinosus insert on the tibia at the inside of the knee.

THE LOWER LEG These are the muscles that straighten or turn up the foot and toes. They are located at the front of the leg and foot.

The extensors The tibialis anterior is the main muscle for pulling up the foot. It arises from the front of the tibia and inserts down in the foot. You see its long tendon stand out in front of the ankle when you pull your foot up.

I won't separately describe the other three extensor muscles. While they are weaker than the tibialis anterior, they are important for coordinating movement of the entire foot as you walk.

The calf muscles There are two of these, the gastrocnemius and the soleus.

The gastrocnemius has two heads. It arises at the lower end of the thighbone where this forms two knobby protrusions. The two muscle bellies join about midway down the lower leg and insert into the Achilles tendon, which attaches to the heel. The gastrocnemius works to flex the knee and to flex the foot downward, in opposition to the extensor muscles at the front of the lower leg, which pull the foot upward.

The soleus is located directly underneath the gastrocnemius, but it does not cross the knee joint. Its orgin is on the back of the tibia and head of the fibula. It acts only to flex the foot downward, as when pushing off with each step while walking.

Plantaris This is a small muscle with a relatively minor role in flexing the knee and foot. It arises on the outside lower "knob" of the thighbone and inserts via a long skinny tendon into the Achilles tendon. While it is not a significant muscle in terms of strength or development as a bodybuilder, it can be a source of trouble if the tendon ruptures. That will prevent an athlete from running and impede forceful downward flexion of the foot.

These are three muscles along the outside of the lower leg. Two are especially impor- ***The peronei*** tant. They arise from the fibula—the peroneus longus from the upper two-thirds and the peroneus brevis from the lower two-thirds. They both pass behind the bone that protrudes at the side of the ankle and insert on the outside portion of the foot. The tendon of the peroneus longus continues and also inserts on the inside of the foot. These muscles flex the foot downward and also turn it out to the side. The tendons of these muscles often become inflamed when a person is beginning strenuous activity that calls for a lot of turn- ing or flexion of the foot, as with running or calf raises. They are also important for pro- viding stability in the ankle joint.

This is by no means an exhaustive inventory of the muscles of the body. There are other flexors in the lower leg and foot; there are muscles that lie deeper in the torso; there are others that give stability to the various body joints. It would take many more pages to give a complete listing. However, if you familiarize yourself with those mentioned here, you will have a sense of those that are more important in bodybuilding. Additionally, in working out a routine of exercises to develop those covered here, you will inevitably bring the others into play, also developing them further and contributing to total muscular development.

CORRECT BODY ALIGNMENT—POSTURE

What is good posture and why is it important?

Good posture means that all the body segments are in correct alignment when the body is upright. It is important because it reduces the strain on the muscle groups that with- stand the effects of gravity. (They are sometimes called the antigravity muscles for that very reason.) These are, in particular, the muscles at the back of the hips, the front of the thigh, and the back of the legs (i.e., the gluteals, the quadriceps, and the gastrocnemius and soleus).

Most individuals have poor posture because of poorly developed muscles in the hip and abdominal regions, which results in the hip joint not being properly aligned with the body's center of gravity, and that throws off all the other joints in turn.

To evaluate your posture, you would need to study a full-length photograph of yourself taken from the side while you are looking straight ahead. Or you could have a friend evaluate you as you stand in that same position. A line dropped from a point directly above (the ceiling, for example) should pass directly behind your ear, in front of the shoulder joint, slightly in front of the elbow joint with your arms hanging straight down, directly "through" the hip joint, and in front of the knee and ankle joints on its way to the floor. If it doesn't, adjust your posture accordingly.

If you do not practice good posture habits, you will find that your body begins to assume a habitual slump or slouch. You risk strain or injury to muscles and ligaments, especial- ly in the lower back, when you engage in any strenuous activity. (As a beginning bodybuilder, you'll be at most risk when performing squats or lunges.) Even if you suc- ceed in developing your musculature beyond that of the average individual, you will not achieve the overall image of vitality and good form that is potentially yours.

The value of good posture can be reflected in your general health picture as well as in relation to a physical activity program. Poor posture means poor alignment of the spinal column. This bony column houses the spinal cord, which gives off a pair of nerves be- tween each pair of vertebrae. These nerves lead to and control all the muscles and organs **21**

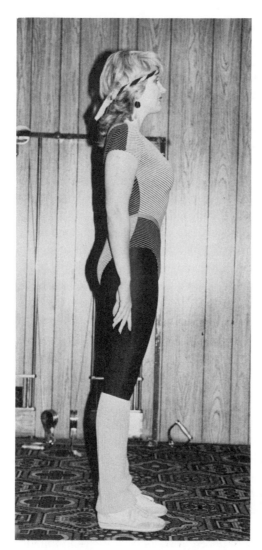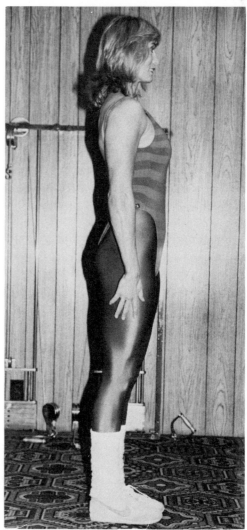

Although Terry Doyle and I have different body types, correct posture makes it possible for both of us to show off our physiques to best advantage. Note how the alignment is almost exactly the same for both of us.

of the body. If the spinal column is not in proper alignment, the bony vertebrae that compose it can press against these nerves. Even though this may not always lead to acute pain or pathological change, over the long run it can lead to impaired nerve function, which will then translate into the affected muscles and organs functioning at a less than optimum level.

A common example of what happens is the development of menstrual cramps that can be relieved by exercise. During menstruation the uterus is more active than at other times.

In the case of cramps, a woman may adopt a slumped posture in response to the pain. That leads to the muscles of the area being compromised with respect to neurovascular supply. However, if one goes out and runs or exercises during this time, she will notice that the cramps are relieved. The body is forced to adopt better alignment in order to perform the exercise. The cramped muscle groups of the spine are stretched and balance is restored between the muscles, bones, nerves and blood vessels, and the affected internal organs, in this case the uterus.

THE FEMALE FACTOR

While as a bodybuilder understanding your body necessarily means developing an understanding of muscles and muscle action, you must also tune into the effects of being a woman. The lines and build of your body are influenced by sex characteristics. Your sex plays a role in how your body responds to efforts to build it up. And as a female you experience certain phenomena related to the reproductive function.

Menstruation

Every woman, once she passes through adolescence, experiences a regular cycle of ovulation and menstruation under normal conditions—unless, of course, she is pregnant or has passed through menopause. However, it is relatively common to find that young women who engage in strenuous physical activity while maintaining a low level of body fat experience a delay or interruption in that cycle. This is known as amenorrhea, failure to menstruate. It's often seen among dancers, gymnasts, runners, and serious bodybuilders.

I've discovered no evidence that amenorrhea is necessarily a dangerous condition, but it is abnormal in terms of general experience. Many physicians who do not specialize in treating this problem react to it by immediately prescribing hormonal therapy to induce the normal menstrual cycle, but this is really not necessary and can be expensive. To establish or resume the cycle, usually all you need do is gain body weight to a more "natural" level, which generally means some increase in the amount of body fat.

There is some question about whether a woman who is amenorrheic actually ovulates. Until the evidence is more clearcut, I'd advise taking contraceptive precautions even if your menstrual cycle appears to have been interrupted.

As far as normal menstruation is concerned, exercise has been shown to relieve the cramps that affect some women at this time. Certain anti-inflammatory agents like tryptophane offer relief, too, as does a glass of wine in many cases. As a rule, exercise does a better job of offering relief.

Contraception

Many sexually active women, including bodybuilders, rely on oral contraceptives to prevent pregnancy. If you are among them, you should be aware that they influence your hormonal balance and can affect your muscle development, too. Progesterone, contained in virtually all birth control pills, actually promotes some breakdown of muscle tissue. That alone suggests you may do well to look to other contraceptive devices to prevent pregnancy. The estrogen-progesterone combination in the pill can also cause water retention, especially just before the onset of menstruation. This, too, works against you, particularly if you are trying to achieve maximum definition in preparation for an upcoming contest.

Another side effect of the use of birth control pills is the increased risk of developing dangerous blood clots. While these will usually not be of great size, even small blood clots can cause some damage in the liver, kidneys, spleen, or other organs through which blood flows. Large blood clots can cause stroke or heart attacks by impeding or blocking the flow of blood to part of the brain or to the heart respectively. The risk of blood clots increases if you also use a diuretic to flush water from your system, which bodybuilders often do just before a competition, again to enhance muscle definition. Water retained in the system gives a smooth look, which counteracts the impression of muscularity a competition contender wants to give.

Some bodybuilders, women as well as men, rely on anabolic steroids to enhance their muscular potential. That practice exposes them to considerable health risks (see the appendix section on drugs and bodybuilding), and the risks increase if the woman is tak-

23

ing oral contraceptives at the same time. The body's hormonal balance is thrown off that much more. My advice is to stay away from anabolic steroids to begin with. Under no circumstances should you combine them with "the pill."

So where does that leave you with respect to birth control? My advice is to rely on use of a diaphragm. While insertion can sometimes be a bother, it is an effective contraceptive device when correctly used with a spermicidal foam or jelly. I also favor use of intrauterine devices (IUDs), but with these there is sometimes a problem with rejection by the uterus and a very small risk of perforating the uterus, which could require a subsequent hysterectomy.

Pregnancy and Childbirth

A bodybuilder who has been in regular training for some time already previous to becoming pregnant can keep working out. However, she should be very careful to avoid overtraining, as this can lead to oxygen deficiency, which can damage the unborn child. (An out-of-shape woman should avoid hard bodybuilding training altogether once she discovers she's pregnant.)

Many women athletes have been able to continue training into their seventh and eight months of pregnancy. As long as they follow a sensible routine that does not expose them to the dangers of overtraining, this may even provide them a certain advantage. A woman who is in good physical shape will generally have an easier delivery. She can push down harder and deliver more quickly. Also, the self-discipline and self-control that make it possible for her to endure the pain that goes with hard training will help her to endure the pain that accompanies childbirth.

A pregnant women should *never* go into heavy training and dieting in preparation for a contest. There is simply too great a risk of damage to self and/or the unborn child. The heavy training is too stressful. Going on a weight-reduction diet is altogether contrary to the dietary needs that she should be attending to for ensuring healthy growth in the child and maintaining her own health. When it comes to dietary changes, she should follow those recommended for any other woman who is pregnant. Probably an athlete still training while pregnant will need more than the average pregnant non-athlete.

Those bodybuilders who are concerned that pregnancy and childbirth will damage their development potential should take heart from the fact that women bodybuilding champions include many who have won titles after becoming mothers. Make sure to stay in good physical condition during your pregnancy, and you will recover your shape quickly and fully following childbirth.

Menopause

Not much has been done by way of research into the effects of exercise on the menopausal woman. I can only offer you my informed opinion that a regular exercise program—and bodybuilding in particular—is likely to offset many of the negative effects of menopause. Menopause is a time of body deterioration as a result of the natural aging process. Bodybuilding acts to promote tissue growth, so it must counteract deterioration at least to some extent. It will be interesting to see what researchers discover in this area once they turn their attention to it.

KNOW YOUR OWN BODY

The information in this chapter will do much to attune you to the structure and working of your body. However, all this amounts to only an introduction. As a bodybuilder, you have to become sensitive to your body's unique qualities. It's not enough to know what muscles are where and do what. You also have to attend to how your muscles respond to *your* efforts to develop them. You have to recognize that Nature has set limitations on you as well as provided you an amazing potential.

Don't rely only on your mirror to tell you what's happening as you follow your exercise routines. Of course you're working to develop a certain appearance. Or course you'll be checking that in front of a mirror and making adjustments in order to achieve that certain image. But stay in touch with how you feel. You're striving for a condition of optimum health as well as for a particular look. Tune into what your body tells you as you go through your workouts. Learn to distinguish between the pain that indicates a temporary stress on a muscle or muscle group and the pain that announces strain or injury. Be alert for signs that tiredness isn't just a result of a strenuous workout but an indication of a developing health problem.

The information here can help your understanding of your body. However, only by careful attention to your body will you develop the total understanding that enables you safely to achieve your unique potential.

A Health Caution

Before engaging in any strenuous physical activity, particulary if you have been mostly sedentary for five years or more—and also if you are more than thirty years of age— you should consult a physician for a thorough medical checkup. Refer to a physician who is knowledgeable in the area of sports medicine, as he or she will be most qualified to evaluate your ability to carry through with a projected program and best able to treat you if you run into problems with injuries.

The checkup should cover all aspects of your medical history. Your doctor should get a complete rundown on any health problems you've suffered in past years. That includes a review of function in all areas—eyes, ears, nose, and throat; the respiratory system; the circulatory system; the endocrine glands; the gastrointestinal tact; the genito-urinary tract and reproductive organs; blood chemistry; and musculo-skeletal system. There should be a detailed review of possible allergies and of past and current immunizations. You should go over any medications you are taking for whatever reason.

As well as taking a detailed medical history, you should undergo a complete physical exam. This properly entails more than just a quick look in your ears, eyes, nose, and throat, with a brief listen to your heart and lungs and a couple of routine blood samples being drawn.

A thorough physical exam should include the following:

- Monitoring of body temperature, pulse, and blood pressure in both arms and both legs, seated and standing
- A weight check
- Examination of any skin lesions or abnormalities
- A vision check and eye examination
- Close examination of the nose, throat, and mouth, including a look at your teeth
- Palpations of the neck, particularly the thyroid
- Inspection of all the lymph nodes that can be palpated from the surface—in the front and back of the neck, in the armpits, and in the groin

- Stethoscopic examination of the heart and lung action, including percussion of the chest and check of the great vessels in the neck, stomach, and groin areas
- A breast examination
- A check of the feet and ankles for any indication of swelling
- Palpation of the calves to check for pain and increased temperature
- An abdominal check by stethoscope, with palpation to check for lumps and percussion to determine the presence of any unusual mass
- Palpation of the liver
- A Pap smear
- A stool examination
- Test of the joints—shoulders, knees, ankles, hips—for possible ligamentous instability—or limited range of movement
- Test of reflexes at the knees, elbows, and behind the heel
- Evaluation of major muscle groups for any weakness or loss of range of motion
- A neurological rundown—checking memory, sense of smell, visual acuity, corneal reflex, gag reflex, balance, and heel-to-toe walking

Depending on what these elements of examination reveal, there may or may not be a need for further tests. A stress electrocardiogram is recommended for anyone who has not engaged in strenuous activity for more than five years, who has a family history of heart disease, or who has elevated blood pressure levels.

Blood tests should be done to determine blood counts and concentrations of red cells and white cells, type of cells, hemoglobin levels, blood sugar levels, and the amounts of other blood components—protein, albumin, calcium, phosphorous, cholesterol, uric acid, total bilirubin, alkaline phosphatase, and other enzymes affecting function of the internal organs.

If you have not had a chest x ray done in the past year, one should be taken now.

This complete physical workup is your best guard against unexpectedly being caught by a health problem when you undertake weight training. You'll be able to proceed confidently, without having to worry that there's risk of damage as a result of the increased heavy physical activity characteristic of bodybuilding.

You should, however, recognize that there is always some risk of injury in any intense physical activity. In the unlikely event that you do incur a training injury, there are steps you can take to minimize its severity.

If the injury is minor, you need only rest the affected body part for one or two workouts and then train it with relatively light weights for the first two or three workouts thereafter.

More serious injuries should first be iced down to prevent swelling and the slower recovery time that results from such swelling. You can simply rub an ice cube over the injured muscle or joint in a circular motion. Or you can fill a plastic bag with ice cubes and a little water and hold that over the injured area.

Any disabling injury—and this includes those occasioning persistent pain or restricted motion—should immediately be checked by a physician. And then you should follow his or her recommendations to the letter. Other injuries can be iced periodically for twenty-four hours after the injury occurred, perhaps ten minutes every three or four hours. Next the injured area should be totally rested for two days, after which you can commence gentle range of motion combined with alternating ice and warm whirlpool treatments.

For more information on dealing with sports injuries, refer to the sports medicine book cited in the bibliography. See also the comments on pages 59–60 (on developing a training instinct) and pages 69–70 (on overtraining) in this book.

YOUR BODY'S NUTRITIONAL NEEDS | 2

There is no one pattern of diet that is perfect for everyone. There is no one food item that is absolutely essential for good health. However, there are several food groups and a host of specific nutrients contained in those that are essential to good health. We do require a certain number of calories and specific fatty acids, amino acids, vitamins, minerals, and trace elements in sufficient amounts and proper combination for growth, maintenance, and repair of body tissues.

Individual needs vary. The standards established by national or international health agencies cannot be applied absolutely to every individual—they are far too general. Also, they only provide guidelines for the average individual, and bodybuilders are not average in terms of nutrition needs.

Bodybuilding requires close attention to personal patterns of food consumption and resultant physical development. You really have to design your own nutrition program. In order to do so, you have to develop an understanding of your body's nutritional needs.

There are six elements of importance in a bodybuilder's diet—protein, carbohydrates, fats, vitamins, minerals, and water. These elements in the right combination contribute to the development of a strong, muscular physique. Where a proper balance is not struck between them, the end result can be an underweight or overweight condition or, in cases of extreme imbalance or deficiency, poor health.

The guidelines in this chapter should be sufficient to orient you to diet choices compatible with the bodybuilding lifestyle. You should realize, however, that it's impossible to go into all the details in a book of this scope. As you feel the need for more information, refer to any of the excellent nutrition guides listed in the bibliography at the end of this book.

For now, let's quickly review the six food elements in the context of your needs as a bodybuilder. We'll move from the least controversial to the most argued food element in our sequence of review.

WATER

Most bodybuilders don't give water a second thought. They should! Your body is largely composed of water; besides that, water acts as an important cleansing agent in the body.

Hard weight training demands a relatively high protein diet for best results. As protein is metabolized in the body, it breaks down into various waste products that must be filtered from the bloodstream through the kidneys and eliminated via the urinary tract. This is true of waste products from carbohydrate and fat metabolism as well, but the waste products of protein metabolism are potentially more dangerous. If a sufficient amount of water isn't taken in to help flush these wastes through, they may form kidney stones. Bodybuilders I've known who have suffered from kidney stones say that it is a fate almost worse than death.

So you must drink water—at least eight to ten glasses a day. That will provide you enough to maintain the proper water composition of your body and to flush through the wastes you must eliminate.

A problem arises in that many municipal water systems serve you water that includes toxic chemicals and sometimes even pollutants. The obvious solution is to drink purified water. In many areas, you can get purified water delivered to your home in large multigallon bottles. Otherwise, you can usually find purified water sold in gallon jugs at your supermarket.

Avoid buying purified water that has had various minerals "added for taste." These minerals have generally not been chelated (bonded to protein molecules), so they are not readily used by the body. That means they just add to the work load on your kidneys.

Note that consumption of liquids other than water is not the same as drinking water. Pure water cleanses by flushing out your system. Other liquids actually introduce new toxins and wastes to your system. Coffee and tea add caffeine and acids as well as their water content. Sodas add sugar—or, in the case of diet sodas, artificial sweeteners—and chemical preservatives. Fruit juices add sugar and some acidity. The best course to follow with liquid intake is to drink pure water as much as possible.

VITAMINS

Vitamins are a popular subject among bodybuilders. Sometimes they are credited with almost magical properties, and many people assume that they are among the good things that you can't get too much of. And so it is that you find bodybuilders taking megadoses of vitamin supplements in order to ensure themselves of all the benefits possible.

Vitamins are essential nutrients. The body requires them in order to function properly. The question then is not really whether they are a necessary part of your diet, but whether supplementation is necessary and, if so, how much of what when.

While the Food and Drug Administration insists that the normal American diet will provide you with your minimum vitamin requirements, I say don't count on it. If all your food could be eaten fresh and in proper proportions, it *might* be possible to consume sufficient vitamins. Unfortunately, in today's world there are very few genuinely fresh foods available. Even so-called fresh vegetables and fruits have usually been transported hundreds or thousands of miles over the course of several days during which vitamins break down and are lost. When a fruit or vegetable has been frozen, it loses a lot of vitamins merely in the oxidation process that occurs as it thaws. Cooking also destroys some vitamins, adding to the potential for vitamin deficiency in the average diet.

To see which supplemental vitamins you might need and why you need them, let's briefly run down the list.

Vitamin A is a fat-soluble vitamin needed for healthy skin and good vision. It also helps fight infection and is valuable to proper growth and development in children. You can obtain it from both animal and vegetable sources. The most common animal source is fish liver oil, and most supplemental vitamin A is derived from shark or cod liver oil. Vegetables do not contain vitamin A as such, but contain concentrations of carotene, which the body easily converts into vitamin A.

The FDA recommends about 5000 international units (I.U.) of vitamin A daily for normally sedentary adults. Certainly bodybuilders will need somewhat greater amounts. However, taking too much vitamin A can result in hypervitaminosis A, a state of toxicity. This has been seen among food faddists who take megadoses of vitamin A in the range of twenty to thirty times the recommended daily allowance (U.S.R.D.A.) over an extended period of time. Your body can store vitamin A, so excessive intake can accumulate to potentially dangerous levels. The usual symptoms of hypervitaminosis A are itching and scaling of the skin, hair loss, and painful swellings of bone tissue.

Common dietary sources of vitamin A besides fish liver oil and yellow, orange, or red vegetables are butter, whole milk, and eggs. Except for liver, meats have only trace amounts of vitamin A.

The B-complex vitamins are all water-soluble and cannot be stored in the body. It is important therefore to consume them in sufficient quantity on a daily basis, if not actually several times per day. As with vitamin A, the B-complex vitamins are obtainable both through animal (mainly meat) and vegetable (mainly brewer's yeast) sources.

There is a wide variety of B-complex vitamins, and it's helpful to have a sense of what each contributes to your health.

Vitamin B-1 (thiamine) is important for muscle growth and for proper utilization of carbohydrates taken in as fuel for energy. There are no toxic effects known in connection with megadoses of thiamine. Beriberi is a disease resulting from thiamine deficiency. Good natural sources of thiamine are whole grains (white flour and polished rice are practically devoid of thiamine unless commercially enriched), brewer's yeast, and pork. The recommended daily allowance is 0.5 mg. (micrograms) per 1000 calories of intake for young adults and 1.0 mg. per 1000 calories for older persons.

Vitamin B-2 (riboflavin) is necessary for normal cellular respiration. Many nutritionists believe riboflavin deficiency to be the most common nutritional deficiency in modern America. Symptoms of deficiency include skin problems, fissures and cracking at the sides of the mouth, and uncomfortable sensitivity of the eyes to light. You may become riboflavin deficient if you omit dairy foods and animal protein from your diet. Good sources of this vitamin are organ meats, cheese, milk, eggs, and brewer's yeast. The recommended daily allowance for adults is from 1.3 to 1.7 mg.

Vitamin B-3 (niacin) is important for enzyme production in your body. Without niacin you would develop digestive tract and nervous system disorders. Brewer's yeast, wheat germ, peanuts, and liver are all good natural sources. If you take certain types of niacin tablets, you will experience an itchy flush in your face and neck shortly afterward. This is not harmful and lasts only a short while. If large doses of niacin are taken for prolonged periods, there is a possibility of irritation of the digestive tract and liver damage. The dosage in that case would be several grams per day. The U.S.R.D.A. is about 20 mg. for the average adult.

Vitamin B-6 (pyridoxine) is essential in human nutrition. It is important for maintaining a balanced body chemistry and plays an important role in protein metabolism. Deficiency can result in skin disorders, weight loss, and neurological disorders such as irritability, confusion, and loss of a sense of responsibility; there may be increased susceptibility to certain types of infections. Women taking oral contraceptives generally require extra B-6 to prevent deficiency. The U.S.R.D.A. is 2.0 mg. for the average adult, 2.5 mg. for pregnant and lactating women. If daily protein intake is more than 100 grams, a greater amount of B-6 will be needed. This is a common situation for bodybuilders.

Vitamin B-6 occurs naturally in meat, cereals, lentils, nuts, and some vegetables and fruits, especially bananas and avocados. There are no known serious toxic effects from megadoses of this vitamin.

Vitamin B-12 (cyanocobalamin) is an essential nutrient for all cells in the body. It's particularly important in maintaining a balanced blood chemistry. Deficiency can lead to pernicious anemia and to neurologic disorders such as loss of sensation. The risk of deficiency is run primarily by individuals (vegans) who eat no animal products whatsoever.

The recommended dietary allowance for normal adults is 10 to 15 mg. It is higher for pregnant or lactating women, and bodybuilders will require even higher amounts, possibly as much as 30 mg. per day. Some people believe B-12 injections to be particularly beneficial, but there's no evidence to indicate a superior benefit. There is danger of scarring of superficial tissues as a result of repeated injections.

Liver is the best source of Vitamin B-12; it is also found in milk and egg yolks.

Vitamin B-15 (pangamic acid) and **vitamin B-17 (laetrile)** are not considered true B-complex vitamins, although sometimes touted as such by health food outlets. There's no evidence of need for or benefit from either. Laetrile, a fad nostrum for certain cancers, may in fact have a toxic effect on the body.

Biotin is a B-complex vitamin important for normal growth and maintenance of health. Deficiency may impair the body's ability to regulate cholesterol levels. The average American diet provides from 100 to 300 mg. of biotin per day. Avidin, a protein contained in egg white, can interfere with biotin absorption unless inactivated by cooking. Bodybuilders who consume raw eggs should take note. Organ meats, soybeans, rice, bran, and egg yolk contain the most biotin, with lesser quantities in dairy products, meats, grains, fruits, and vegetables.

Choline, another B-complex vitamin, is common in many foods, too, and there is no evidence of dietary deficiency. Bodybuilders often take it supplementally because of its reputed value in speeding metabolism of body fat, which has not been definitely confirmed by medical research. It's found mostly in egg yolks, organ meats, grains, and legumes. Fruits and vegetables are a poorer source.

Inositol, also a B-complex vitamin, is credited with the same fat-metabolizing powers as choline. Again, that property has not been confirmed by medical research. Inositol is widely abundant in all foods; a normal diet will provide from 300 to 1000 mg. per day. There's no evidence of toxic effect with consumption of megadoses over short periods of time.

Folic acid (folate) is an important B-complex nutrient. Deficiency can lead to certain forms of anemia. Alcohol apparently interferes with the body's use of folate. Certain drugs do as well, including oral contraceptives. Supplemental quantities of folic acid are therefore recommended for women taking oral contraceptives, together with supplemental B-12, which is closely associated with folic acid in the body. The U.S.R.D.A. is 400 mg. for the average adult, boosted to 600 to 800 mg. for pregnant or lactating women.

Folic acid is contained mostly in liver, dark green leafy vegetables, lima beans, kidneys, nuts, whole grain cereals, and lentils. It is also produced in the intestine itself, so that deficiency is unusual.

Para-amino-benzoic acid (PABA) acts in concert with many of the other B-complex vitamins to keep normal body functions on an even keel. Good natural sources include milk, brewer's yeast, liver, eggs, rice bran, and wheat germ.

Vitamin C, like the B-complex vitamins listed above, is water-soluble and cannot be stored in the body. It is vitally necessary for cell integrity, for maintaining the health and strength of connective tissue, as a natural agent preventing bruising and promoting healing, and as a cleansing agent in the body. A serious deficiency will lead to scurvy. On a less serious level, with insufficient intake of vitamin C, you will find it difficult to recover quickly from your strenuous workouts.

The U.S.R.D.A. is 50 mg. for the average adult and 60 mg. for pregnant and lactating women. During periods of increased physical stress, as with bodybuilding training, it's required in greater quantities.

Vitamin C is largely destroyed in the cooking process. Prolonged standing at room temperature will also result in vitamin C loss. Freezing, on the other hand, does not seem to result in a loss. Smoking, aspirin use, and use of oral contraceptives all reduce vitamin C blood levels.

Citrus fruits are prime sources for vitamin C, as are other raw or minimally cooked fresh fruits and vegetables. Megadoses are said by some to increase resistance to infections such as the common cold. There's no known toxic effect from megadoses, although certain types of kidney stones may result from increased excretion of compounds known as oxalates stimulated by massive vitamin C doses. If you use supplemental vitamin C, it makes no difference if it's from rose hips, acerola berries, green peppers or manufactured.

Vitamin D is fat-soluble, like vitamin A. It plays an important role in calcium metabolism, ensuring strong, healthy bones and teeth. Again, fish liver oils are the best natural source of vitamin D, although if you spend much time in the sun, the action of the sun will stimulate production of vitamin D in the skin, eliminating any need for supplementation. Excessive intake of over 100,000 I.U. to 200,000 I.U. per day may result in abnormally high levels of calcium in the blood, with risk of damage to the heart and major arteries and kidneys. Never take more than 1,000 I.U. per day without a physician's supervision.

Vitamin D deficiency can lead to loss of calcium from the bones, with subsequent skeletal weakness. This problem occurs most with women who have avoided milk and other dietary sources of calcium and vitamin D out of fears about gaining weight. Vitamin D is also important for building muscle strength, which can be compromised by a dietary deficiency.

Vitamin E, another fat-soluble nutrient, has become one of the most popular food supplements among bodybuilders. It is promoted for cardiac and vascular health and as an aid in increasing workout endurance. It is believed by many to retard the body deterioration evident in aging. The average nutritional requirement is about 15 mg. per day.

Scientists have formulated a synthetic vitamin E, but most health-oriented nutritionists recommend choosing the naturally derived supplement. Acetate E is the synthetic form. The D-alpha tocopherol component is the most important, but you may want capsules labeled "mixed tocopherols." Wheat germ oil is the best natural source of unrefined vitamin E.

Vitamin F is another fat-soluble vitamin. Its effect in the body has not yet been isolated. It is supplied in the diet by unsaturated fats.

Vitamin K, also a fat-soluble vitamin, plays an important role in the chemistry of blood clotting. A deficiency can lead to an increased bleeding tendency. Use of antibiotic drugs may lead to a deficiency, since this vitamin is also produced in the intestine by beneficial microorganisms that are destroyed by the antibiotic action.

The U.S.R.D.A. for vitamin K is not known. It is probably in the area of 1 to 2 mg. per kilogram of body weight per day. The average diet contains from 300 to 400 mg. per day, so a person in normal health eating a balanced diet should be getting more than enough. Vitamin K is abundant in green leafy vegetables.

Bioflavonoids are a group of compounds widely distributed in plants, where they act to protect ascorbic acid (vitamin C) and other plant components from oxidation. They are concentrated in the skin or peel of fruits and vegetables. Tea, coffee, wine, and beer contain large amounts of bioflavonoids, as does the white inner skin of citrus fruits. Some nutritionists point to the bioflavonoids' close association with vitamin C as an indication of their importance, but medical research has yet to confirm a necessary role for them in the human body. Lack of evidence for a necessary role in the diet leads to some question about whether bioflavonoids are properly termed vitamins, even though in years past they were collectively identified as vitamin P.

VITAMIN SUPPLEMENTS

Women taking oral contraceptives will probably require supplementation of vitamin B-6, folic acid, vitamin B-12, and vitamin C.

The hard training of bodybuilding will also lead to a likely need for supplementation because of the associated increase in metabolism. Also, there may be increased nutrient loss through sweat or urine.

Some bodybuilders rely on vitamin and mineral supplements to such an extent that they spend up to $500 per month for them prior to an important competition. That is obviously not practical for most of us.

I recommend purchasing vitamin and mineral "multipacks," one of which will provide at least the amount of vitamins, minerals, and trace elements that you need each day. You should take at least one multipack per day. Most champion bodybuilders take two or three per day, usually with their meals to promote better assimilation in the digestive tract. Multipacks are produced by many health food companies, and the average retail price for a cellophane packet of tablets is about 50¢.

Then I recommend that you try vitamin B-complex tablets or capsules, since it is difficult to build muscle mass without adequate supplies of B-complex in your diet.

After that, in descending order of importance (based on my experience as a physician and athlete), try individual supplements of vitamin C, vitamin E, pantothenic acid, vitamin A, vitamin D, choline, inositol, vitamin B-12, and PABA. (See also the comments on mineral supplements on page 35.)

MINERALS

Like vitamins, minerals are absolutely vital to your health. They help to build body structure and coordinate the body's metabolic processes.

The most important minerals for bodybuilders are calcium, phosphorous, magnesium, potassium, sodium, chlorine, sulfur, iron, copper, iodine, fluorine, manganese, and zinc. There is a lab test that many physicians can give you to determine whether you are consuming minerals in sufficient quantity for optimum health. The test involves analysis of a hair sample to determine mineral concentrations.

Let's run down the list of minerals to see what's important about each one.

Calcium is mostly concentrated in the skeleton and is important for a healthy bone structure. However, the small amount of calcium that does not go into bone formation is equally essential. It acts in concert with phosphorous and vitamins A, C, and D to ensure proper physiological balance. Among vital functions affected are the heart's pumping action, the activation of digestive enzymes, blood clotting, the regulation of fluid passing through cell walls, and proper nerve transmission.

Most young and middle-aged adults can stay in positive calcium balance with an average daily intake of 1000 mg. per day. That balance is negatively affected by diets that are high in phosphorous (such as meats and soft drinks), and the imbalance can lead to calcium loss, weakening the skeleton.

Calcium supplements are extremely important to bodybuilders who are dieting for a competition, because most precontest diets are relatively low in the mineral. Meats are high in phosphorous, and milk products, which are high in calcium, are often eliminated during contest preparation. As calcium levels in the blood drop, one tends to become nervous and irritable, which some nutritionists term the "phosphorous jitters," because of the characteristic imbalance between calcium and phosphorous.

The calcium balance is also negatively influenced by a number of other practices indulged in by some bodybuilders. Those who use diuretics to achieve definition at contest time promote rapid calcium loss that can cause muscle cramps. (Dyazide is one such diuretic.) The practices of carbohydrate loading, high protein diet, and taking thyroid and growth hormone substances can also promote calcium excretion, so bodybuilders who engage in any of these should be aware of a likely need for supplementation. An intake ranging from 1000 to 2500 mg. per day is generally safe. Taking calcium supplements in larger amounts could result in kidney stones because of hypercalcemia, excessive concentrations of calcium in the bloodstream.

Phosphorous acts in complement with calcium. It is essential for proper function in the transmission of nerve impulses, muscle contraction, fat and carbohydrate metabolism, hormone secretion, and mental alertness. It is an important component of bone tissue.

The U.S.R.D.A. for phosphorous is the same as that for calcium, in order to maintain balance between the two. Milk, poultry, fish, and meat are major sources. Non-nutritious soft drinks contain excessive phosphorous in the form of phosphoric acid. While there is no demonstrated toxic effect from excessive amounts of phosphorous, there is an effect relative to calcium balance. Maintaining a phosphorous-calcium balance is important, as we've noted above.

Magnesium plays an important role as a coenzyme to build protein within the body. It is also a factor in healthy muscle action.

It is difficult to establish accurate dietary requirements because of magnesium's complex interaction with other nutrients. The usual recommendations are for 300 to 400 mg. per day for adults. An overabundance is not a problem as long as kidney function is normal.

Good natural sources include sunflower seeds, beet tops, cucumbers, cauliflower, figs, grapefruit, and vegetable oils.

Potassium is essential for maintenance of a correct water balance in the body and for the prevention of muscle cramps. A potassium deficiency can make you feel weak and lacking in energy during a workout. Diuretic abuse contributes seriously to dangerous potassium deficiency states.

Natural sources of potassium include grapefruit, bananas, and green peppers.

Sodium also helps maintain the body's vital water balance. It has a high affinity for water, so during the last *few days* prior to competition, you should avoid consuming sodium or you will find it hard to achieve good definition. Too much water in your system will smooth out your muscularity. Avoid sugarless diet sodas, as the artificial sweetener is a sodium compound. Cut out table salt in precompetition, too, as it is also a sodium compound. The average American diet contains more than enough sodium, so supplementation is rarely a consideration.

Chlorine is important to the production of digestive acids and for elimination of wastes from the body. Bodybuilders value its contribution to tendon, ligament, and cartilage health. Kelp, dulse, ripe olives, and green leafy vegetables are good natural sources of chlorine.

Sulfur helps to keep your hair, fingernails, and skin healthy-looking. It plays a vital role in the body's production of amino acids, which we'll discuss in a moment. Eggs, fish, cabbage, and brussels sprouts are good natural sources.

Iron is an essential component of the red blood cells, which accomplish oxygen transfer within the body. Men and nonmenstruating women in good health require from 12 to 18 mg. per day. Menstruating women will require more, perhaps as much as 23 mg. per day, and pregnant women as much as 35 mg. per day.

The average American diet provides between 10 to 30 mg. per day. However, a weight-conscious woman limiting caloric intake to between 1000 and 1500 calories per day will probably take in only from 6 to 9 mg., so supplementation is advised, and also for menstruating and pregnant women. Ferrous iron is the more easily absorbed form, although the body can also use ferric iron.

Iron deficiency most commonly leads to iron deficiency anemia, a condition characterized by easy tiring, vague irritability, and increased susceptibility to infection. An iron overload can result in tissue damage. The deficiency state is more common—almost 50 percent of all young women have some degree of iron deficiency anemia. The danger of overload is sufficiently great that you should not take more than the recommended daily allowance for your sex and physiological state.

Good natural sources are eggs, raisins, molasses, cherries, plums, and green leafy vegetables.

Copper also plays a vital role in the blood transport of oxygen. It is required for incorporation of iron into the hemoglobin of red blood cells. Dried beans, almonds, prunes, whole wheat, and peas are good natural sources. Copper is also present in the amino acid tyrosine.

Iodine helps regulate body metabolism. Many bodybuilders believe it stimulates the thyroid gland, thereby speeding up metabolism to burn off fat. So they take kelp tablets, which have a high iodine content, to aid in cutting up before a contest. Note, however, that before 1943 physicians used to treat hyperthyroidism (overactive thyroid) by administering Lugol's solution, which is a concentrate of potassium iodide. If iodine in this form slows metabolism, it may be that taking kelp tablets actually impedes efforts to cut up.

Manganese interacts with B-complex vitamins to provide the benefits they offer and also helps to build strong joints and bones. It is found in eggs, peas, sunflower seeds, and green leafy vegetables.

Zinc is involved in insulin production, energy production, and vitamin metabolism. You will get enough zinc if you eat liver regularly, or you can use supplemental tablets.

Fluorine is probably the least important dietary mineral for bodybuilders. Minute amounts help strengthen the teeth. You will get enough for your bodily needs simply by

following a normally balanced diet.

When you take supplemental minerals, it is essential that they be *chelated*. Chelation is a chemical process in which protein molecules are bonded to molecules of a mineral. Chelation is vital, because it transforms minerals from an inorganic form that cannot be used in the body to organic substances that can be utilized.

The minerals you are most likely to need in supplemental form are iron, potassium, calcium, manganese, and magnesium. These supplements should be taken in combination with vitamin supplements and protein supplements you may be using to balance your nutritional needs. (See page 32.) You may also want to take dessicated liver as a food supplement because of its diverse vitamin and mineral content.

FATS

Fats, also known as lipids, are very high in energy—9 kilocalories per gram, compared to the 4 kilocalories contained in a gram of either protein or carbohydrate. Fats are made up of chains of fatty acids, and there is a whole range of possible combinations from what are called short-chain fatty acids to long-chain fatty acids. Depending on their chemical composition, they are either unsaturated or saturated. (The distinction lies in whether the fatty acids are so linked that all the molecular binding sites are used or not.) The shorter and more unsaturated a fatty acid chain is, the more likely the resultant fat will be liquid or soft at room temperature. The longer and more saturated fatty acid chain will be more solid. In the refining process called hydrogenation, food processors transform shorter, unsaturated fats into longer, more saturated (and hence harder) fats. Margarine and shortening are two produced by hydrogenation of vegetable fats, which are naturally more liquid.

Except for coconut oil, which is almost completely saturated (and rich in vitamin E), vegetable oils are generally unsaturated. Animal fats are more saturated than vegetable fats, but vary among themselves. The fat in beef or mutton is more saturated than the fat of pork or poultry. (I used to take it for granted that pork fat was the most saturated.) Fat from fish is softer and less saturated than that from beef, mutton, pork, or poultry.

Fats are probably the biggest problem with the average American diet, particularly excessive intake of animal fats. Fat makes up about 42 percent of the average American diet. The essential fatty acid requirement amounts to only 2 to 3 percent of one's total caloric intake, but most dietitians agree that a 25 percent proportion of the diet is best for maintaining the taste quality of foods and satisfying hunger cravings.

Some people believe that any fat in the diet should be avoided when it comes to holding weight down; but that is a misconception. For one thing, fat provides an excellent source of energy that can be stored for necessary use later. You do need energy stores in order to meet the demands of exhaustive workouts and the extra stresses that are not necessarily a part of average life routines. The point is to avoid storing too much, not to avoid storing any at all. Fat will also decrease the amount of protein you lose when your body has to manufacture its own glucose from noncarbohydrate sources, as happens with low-carbohydrate diets. (More on that later.)

Fat in the body also protects body organs and nerves against trauma, providing a sort of padding effect. This can be very important for athletes, who probably subject their internal organs to more trauma than nonathletes. Fat acts as an insulator for maintaining body temperatures, although athletes, who are highly active, will not want so much insulation that they can't disperse the rapid buildup in body heat that comes with strenuous activity.

Fat is important in the transport and absorption of the fat-soluble vitamins, which are essential to good health. Fat reduces the body's need for thiamine as part of the process for metabolizing carbohydrates. In the absence of sufficient supplies of the two known essential fatty acids, linoleic and arachidonic, there can be a breakdown in the integrity of cell membranes. This can be reflected in poor skin quality and tendency to injuries like tendinitis and bursitis. I've observed a lot of athletes with very low levels of body fat chronically plagued by injuries like these.

Strange as it may seem, fats play an important role in appetite control. They provide you a satisfied feeling after a meal; they slow the emptying of the stomach so that you don't feel impelled to eat again as soon as you otherwise might.

Fat is of particular concern to bodybuilders, because just a little "too much" of it masks muscle definition. The bodybuilder will have a smooth or soft appearance, which will count against her when it comes to assessing muscle development. Monitoring fat intake rather than eliminating it altogether, exposing you to possible negative side effects, is usually the answer. An easy weight gainer should eliminate most of the fat from her diet. If you happen to be of average build and metabolism, it's all right to eat a little fat, but probably less than you do eat. If your are a hard gainer, eat the fats that naturally occur in your diet, but don't go out of your way to consume more.

FATS AND CHOLESTEROL

Cholesterol, much talked about in connection with cardiovascular illness, is an essential food substance. A member of the alcohol family, it is found primarily in animal products. It is necessary for the health and proper functioning of cell membranes and brain and nerve tissue. It is very important in the production of natural steroid hormones. It is essential for the proper absorption of fat. It plays a part in vitamin D metabolism. It gives the skin resistance to a host of chemical agents that would otherwise prove irritants.

The difficulty arises with excessive levels of cholesterol in the blood. Diets that are high in fat—in particular, diets high in saturated fats—produce high serum cholesterol levels. High serum cholesterol levels are associated with atherosclerosis, hypertension, and diabetes mellitus.

There's much talk of the key being reduction of the amount of cholesterol in the diet, but the fact is that your body itself manufactures more cholesterol than you take in. A high dietary intake of cholesterol of itself actually increases serum cholesterol levels by only a few points. However, a diet very high in saturated fats can increase serum cholesterol levels from 40 to 50 percent. These fats increase absorption of cholesterol and stimulate the body to greater production of its own. So the key is really lowering the amount of saturated fats in your diet more than it is lowering cholesterol intake on its own. Animal fats, which are more saturated than vegetable fats, often add a relatively high cholesterol content of their own. Vegetable fats do not in most cases contain cholesterol. Instead, they are high in linoleic acid, which seems to combat cholesterol deposits in the vascular system. Of common vegetable oils, safflower oil is highest in linoleic acid content.

You do not have to make an effort to take in enough linoleic acid, since it is not required in large amounts and is commonly stored in substantial amounts in body tissue. The point is that you'll do better if what fat you do consume is unsaturated and high in linoleic acid, as opposed to being saturated and composed primarily of other fatty acids that allow or encourage high serum cholesterol levels.

36   Because your overall fat needs really are quite low, as a bodybuilder you'll do well to

keep your intake of any of them to a minimum. What oil you do use in cooking should be unsaturated vegetable oils. If you use oil in salad dressings, try to use only safflower oil. Keep your intake of animal fats as low as possible.

CARBOHYDRATES

Carbohydrates, commonly known as sugars and starches, make up 45 to 50 percent of the average American diet. There are many different types of carbohydrates. Most are simple sugars—monosaccharides. Examples of monosaccharides include glucose (known as blood sugar in the body) and fructose (fruit sugar). Two simple sugars combined make up a disaccharide. Sucrose, for example, is a disaccharide made up of fructose and glucose. Several monosaccharides linked together form a polysaccharide. If enough of them link together into a long chain or branched molecule, that polysaccharide is known as a starch.

Carbohydrates are the human body's preferred source of fuel for immediate energy needs, and your body requires a daily supply of them to maintain optimum health and promote proper body function. There are 4 kilocalories per gram of carbohydrate, regardless of the source. It is protein-sparing. Without carbohydrates, your body would convert protein into glucose for energy. You have to have glucose in your diet to prevent breakdown of muscle tissue as a substitute energy source.

Carbohydrate is also necessary for normal fat metabolism. With too little carbohydrate, fat is not oxidized completely. It breaks down into ketones, which create an acidic imbalance in the body. That can lead to sodium combining with acids to form sodium salts, which are then excreted through the urine. There is a danger of severe sodium imbalance; in trying to filter excess sodium from the blood, your kidneys work harder, flushing so much water through that you can become dehydrated.

When people go on a low-carbohydrate diet, they risk fatigue, because the body isn't getting its preferred fuel. They risk kidney damage and the side effects of imbalance in blood chemistry.

In incorporating carbohydrates into your diet, the trick is to establish a balance between them, recognizing the characteristic qualities of the major carbohydrate forms. They are not all metabolized at the same rate of speed. Sugars tend to break down and release energy into the bloodstream very quickly, but you get an energy crash shortly after the initial pickup. Refined carbohydrates, especially white sugar, is the worst for prompting energy rises and falls. They are the main component in most of the so-called junk foods that Americans indulge in with such passion.

The more complex carbohydrates digest more slowly and so release energy more slowly and at a more even level. Rice and other whole grains, potatoes, nuts, seeds, and vegetables are the prime sources for complex carbohydrates.

I suggest you include at least 100 grams of carbohydrate per day in your diet; 150 grams might be even better. Choose carbohydrate foods like fruits and vegetables and whole grain products, which have a high nutritional value including vitamins, minerals, and other nutrients. (While many snack foods are made from grain products, these have usually been stripped of bran and germ layers that contain essential amino acids, vitamins, and minerals. Snack foods commonly include sugar as a main ingredient as well.)

This is not to say that all sugar is to be avoided. Glucose, a simple sugar abundant in fruits, sweet corn, and honey, is an essential body need. Under normal conditions, it's the only energy source the brain can use. In fact, in digestion your body breaks other foods down into glucose (together with lesser amounts of other simple sugars). It passes into the liver, where it is either stored as glycogen or sent out for immediate energy use or storage elsewhere. Excess glucose is converted into fatty acids, forming triglycerides that are stored in fat cells. Balance is important, because some glucose in the liver converts into glucouronic acid, which acts upon toxic chemicals and bacteria so they are properly excreted by the kidneys. So if you deprive yourself of carbohydrates over an extended period of time, you can impair your body's ability to rid itself of toxic wastes, a function dependent on glucose being available in ready quantity.

You cannot depend on glucose stored as glycogen to keep up energy levels during a low-carbohydrate diet period. (Meats are not a good source of glycogen, since it converts into lactic acid in animals at the time of slaughter.) Only a small amount of glycogen is available to the body at any one time, and the body can store only limited amounts in the liver and muscles.

The key to balance is to eat simple sugars in small amounts at regular intervals. Be careful not to eat so much that you wind up building fat. Combine that intake with complex carbohydrates, so energy levels don't fluctuate radically.

Some health faddists draw "important" distinctions between simple sugars that are not always based on a sound understanding of nutrition. Fructose, very plentiful in honey and fruit (like glucose), is a favorite substitute for table sugar (sucrose) among some health-conscious people. The sweetest of sugars, it is two-and-a-half times as sweet as sucrose. The idea is that you'd use less fructose than sucrose, and while this is probably true, it absorbs into the bloodstream as quickly as any sugar. There is no absolute health advantage to using fructose in preference to glucose or sucrose.

Lactose, milk sugar, can provide some people a problem. Some people have a deficiency of lactase, the enzyme required to digest lactose, so they will develop gastrointestinal upset from drinking milk, the most common source of lactose. However, cheese and yogurt contain less lactose than other milk products and may also contain lactase.

Sorbitol is an alcohol derived from glucose. It has the same level of sweetness as glucose, but it is absorbed very slowly, keeping blood sugar levels at a more constant level over longer periods of time. This can be an aid in dieting, because the blood sugar level will stay at a level that delays the onset of hunger feelings as a result of sharp drops in blood sugar.

Corn syrup, an increasingly popular sweetener, is not actually a natural simple sugar, but dextran, the product of a process by which corn starch is broken down into simpler components. Corn syrup is more quickly absorbed than starch, so products with corn sweeteners should also be on your "alert" list when it comes to avoiding energy jags.

Energy jags, of course, are not the whole story when it comes to establishing a proper dietary balance for carbohydrates. A high refined sugar and starch intake has been associated with heart attacks and obesity. Dental caries (cavities) are strongly linked to intake of sugar in any sticky form that leaves the teeth coated.

PROTEIN

The average American consumes about 100 grams of protein per day. The gut is always secreting enzymes and amino acids, too, and this adds another 70 grams per day of protein to the digestive tract. That means the average person absorbs a protein load of approximately 170 grams per day. As protein is the major nonwater component of muscles, as well as of the blood and most other body tissues, establishing a proper protein balance in the body is very important.

The body loses protein every day, too. About 10 grams a day pass through the digestive tract without being absorbed and, on average, about 80 grams are lost via metabolism and excretion through the urinary tract, primarily as nitrogen, the element that is a major component of all proteins. Roughly 2 grams of protein are lost daily through loss of cells in the skin, hair, and nails. That adds up to an average daily loss of from 90 to 100 grams.

Obviously, in order to develop muscle, you have to take in more protein than you lose. So how much do you need? Gauging from studies on the subject, the average person needs about .6 grams per kilogram (1 kilogram equals 2.2 pounds) of body weight. If a high quality protein is consumed, the body can utilize most of the protein available—about 70 percent of the actual protein contained in the food. Whole egg protein is a very high quality protein. The average dietary protein has only about 75 percent of the biological quality of whole egg protein, so that only about 50 percent of the average protein taken in actually gets used by the body. That suggests that people relying primarily on average quality protein sources might do well to calculate a need for .89 grams of protein per kilogram of body weight. But then keep in mind that we're still just talking about the average person, usually described as a 155-pound man with an energy intake just for sufficient maintenance.

Someone engaging in a high-intensity bodybuilding program will need more than the average requirement for sufficient maintenance. She may need as much as 1 to 1.5 grams per kilogram of body weight. For the hard-training competitive bodybuilder, I recommend a diet with a protein content of at least 1.3 grams to 2 grams. It's impossible to be more specific, since individual metabolism requirements vary. Many women bodybuilders consume as little as 40 to 50 grams of protein per day, while others eat more than 200 grams daily. Try varying the amounts and types of protein intake to determine what works best for you.

You should recognize the difference among protein sources. Your body protein contains twenty-two different amino acids. (These are the building blocks making up various proteins.) Eight of these amino acids cannot be produced by the human body itself; they must be taken in through the food you eat. These amino acids—histidine, isolucine, leucine, lysine, methionine, phenylalanine, threonine, tryptophan, and valine—are termed *essential*. The other amino acids are just as necessary for health and growth, but they can be produced in the body itself from substances present in the average diet. They are nonessential, in the sense that they needn't be present in final form in what you eat.

The essential amino acids are present in sufficient quantities in all animal-source protein—meat, eggs, dairy products, fish. In contrast, vegetable proteins either totally lack one or more essential amino acid or have very low concentrations of them. Researchers have calculated what they call the protein efficiency ration (PER) for most foods. Generally speaking, the higher the essential amino acid content of a protein food, the higher its PER. Animal-source proteins have a much higher PER than proteins from vegetable sources. Biologically, the best protein sources are egg whites, fish, milk products, poultry, and red meats. By thoughtfully combining vegetable and/or animal proteins in a meal, however, you can improve the relative PER of each food within the combination. Here are three good protein food combinations:

1. Rice + beans
2. Corn + beans or lentils
3. Milk + corn, beans, lentils, or rice

When protein is taken in in the diet, it is broken down and absorbed through the intestinal wall as amino acids. The amino acids are then transported to the liver and distributed from there to serve their various vital functions. Of the amino acids absorbed, from 20 to 40 percent (depending on individual metabolism and activity levels) goes to the repair and growth of muscles. So the significance of protein for bodybuilders is obvious.

But it's not as simple as merely eating enough protein, even in the right combination to ensure getting the essential amino acids. You also have to take into account your body's ability to absorb the protein you take in. The average person can only digest and assimilate about 30 grams of protein per meal, so eating 100 grams at a meal doesn't automatically increase the amount available in your bloodstream.

You can make more protein available for assimilation into muscle tissue if you consume small meals five or six times a day rather than large meals two or three times each day. Smaller meals are more easily digested, and the more frequent meals add to the amount of digested protein available for muscle growth. Taking this into account, here is a sample weight-gain menu you can use when in heavy training to increase the size of your muscles:

Meal One (7:00 A.M.)—three soft-boiled eggs, a slice of whole-grain toast, a glass of milk, supplements
Meal Two (9:30 A.M.)—protein drink
Meal Three (12:00 noon)—tuna salad, piece of fruit, a glass of milk, supplements
Meal Four (2:30 P.M.)—protein drink
Meal Five (5:00 P.M.)—broiled chicken, rice, green or yellow vegetables, a glass of milk, supplements
Meal Six (8:00 P.M.)—cold cuts, hard-boiled eggs, milk, supplements

For your protein drink, here is a good recipe you can quickly mix up in a blender:

8 to 10 oz. of milk
1 to 2 tablespoons of milk and egg protein
soft fruit for flavoring (bananas, strawberries, peaches, etc.)

If you are slightly allergic to milk—your stomach bloats after drinking it—substitute a fruit juice or iced tea to drink your protein concentrate in. If you want to consume milk products for their protein value, you will find you can eat yogurt and hard cheeses, as these have very low lactose levels. The general rule of thumb is to eat 2 or 3 ounces of cheese for each glass of milk you'd otherwise drink. Yogurt, a cultured milk product, has less lactose than whole milk, while containing more lactase. That makes it a valuable source of dietary calcium for people with a lactase deficiency. (Lactase is an enzyme that aids in the digestion of certain food substances.)

Bodybuilders sometimes forget the connection that exists between the various food elements, and this is most evident when it comes to devising a diet for reducing body fat. Many bodybuilders like to go on high-protein, low-carbohydrate diets in order to lose fat. However, when they do, they also end up losing muscle (which on average forms 45 percent of body weight), because carbohydrates play a role in building up muscle tissue from amino acids in dietary protein. This happens through the mechanism of insulin transport. Insulin will only be present if carbohydrates have been taken in, because that is what stimulates insulin production. Amino acids are carried into muscle cells by insulin. If you do not have carbohydrate in your reducing diet, you will not only lose fat, you will reduce muscle, too.

Keep these basic considerations in mind in planning your protein intake:

- The best protein for bodybuilders and fitness-minded weight trainers come from animal sources. Red meats, however, should be largely avoided because of their high fat content. Eggs, milk products, fish, and poultry are your best animal-protein sources.
- Of the vegetable protein sources, soybeans and sprouted seeds have the best amino acid balances and can be considered fairly good sources of complete protein. However, you need fairly large quantities of vegetable protein to build the same amount of muscle you would attain from eating smaller quantities of the recommended animal-source proteins.
- Keep your protein intake down to about 20 to 30 grams per meal, since your digestive system can't process more than 30 grams per feeding. Eat some complex carbohydrates (vegetables, rice or other grains, potatoes, legumes, seeds and nuts) as well, since this results in more protein being taken up by muscle cells for growth and repair.
- If you take a protein supplement, use it only between meals, or it will go largely wasted (for the reason indicated above). There are three basic types of commercial protein supplements available—meat base, soybean base, and milk-egg base. On a biological value scale, milk-egg protein powder would rate the highest and soya protein the lowest.
- Never drink a liquid amino acid supplement without also taking tryptophan tablets. Liquid amino acids are manufactured from animal by-products in such a way that they are invariably low in the essential amino acid tryptophan.

ROUGHAGE

While roughage—or fiber, as it is commonly called—isn't exactly a nutrient since it isn't digested, it should be part of your diet. It is very important for keeping your digestive tract functioning properly. If you eat large quantities of protein and very little roughage, you will begin to build up protein wastes and residues in your colon. This may eventually cause serious health problems, among them cancer of the colon, the third most frequently occurring type of cancer in the United States.

Roughage also acts as something of a sponge in the gut. It holds water, so that solid wastes do not become so solid as to place strain on the intestine wall, which can lead to a condition called diverticulosis, small hernialike outpouchings of the intestine wall that can easily become irritated or inflamed. Roughage also absorbs bile acids produced in the digestive process, which helps keep blood cholesterol levels down. Retained acids stimulate the production of cholesterol in the body.

You can easily add roughage to your diet without adding calories. Eat bran, plenty of lettuce and celery, and high-roughage fruits like pears. As well as keeping your digestive system healthy, you'll find that the bulk introduced helps control your appetite.

A diet with too much roughage can lead to bezoars forming in the stomach and intestine. (Bezoars are concentrations of vegetable matter such as seeds, skins, and fibers that can obstruct the digestive tract if they become large enough.) However, it isn't all that common a problem, as few people in developed countries take in so much roughage that it overwhelms the system in this way.

VEGETARIANISM

Many champion bodybuilders and other athletes follow vegetarian diets. However, you should understand that there are three vegetarian regimens, and the distinctions are quite meaningful:

1. **Vegans** eat food only from nonanimal sources.
2. **Lacto-vegetarians** add milk products to the nonanimal sources they take in.
3. **Lacto-ovo-vegetarians** will eat eggs as well as milk products in addition to nonanimal foods.

I know of no championship vegan bodybuilders and very few lacto-vegetarians who have won even low-level titles. The overwhelming majority of champion vegetarian bodybuilders are lacto-ovo-vegetarians. If you as a bodybuilder want to follow a vegetarian diet, you will do best to include both milk products and eggs in your diet.

A vegetarian diet can afford you some advantages. Generally speaking, it is relatively low in fat content, which makes it fairly easy to maintain a low level of body fat on a constant basis. Also, vegetarians generally have much greater endurance than those who eat meat. When the digestive system is relieved of the burdensome, energy-consuming task of processing animal fats, the rest of the body benefits from the availability of left-over energy. Since a vegetarian diet contains more roughage, the benefits of that are also yours.

Be alert to possible iron deficiencies and to deficiencies of calcium and zinc in the event you prefer a vegan-type diet. Vegans also lack a natural dietary source of vitamin B-12, since this nutrient comes only from animal sources. Supplements are the answer. You can get extra iron from brewer's yeast, wheat germ, wheat bran, eggs, and enriched flour, as well as from iron supplements available in tablet or capsule form. (Use only deactivated brewer's yeast, to avoid risk of fungal infections that may result from taking live yeast.)

Vegans should avoid a diet depending solely on cereal grains for protein, since many cereals are deficient in lysine, an essential amino acid.

SOME GENERAL DIET TIPS

Here are a number of diet tips that you can apply to supplement the basic guidelines given above. Try each suggestion and use your common sense to determine if it works for you or is particularly applicable to you.

- Good overall dietary goals for someone wishing to have a well-balanced, healthy diet would be to have carbohydrate consumption account for 55 percent of the total calorie intake. The greater part of this should be in the form of complex carbohydrates rather than simple sugars. Reduce overall fat consumption to around 30 percent of the energy intake, and reduce the *saturated* fat consumption to around 10 percent of total energy intake. Keep cholesterol consumption to no more than 200 mg. per day, and limit salt intake to about 3 grams per day. Increase your consumption of fruits, vegetables, and whole grain cereals.

- Avoid drinking calories. You can drink 1000 calories of orange juice in one-tenth the time it would take you to eat 1000 calories of whole oranges.
- Many people are mildly allergic to grains and/or milk products. If either of these food groups tends to bloat your body, be particularly careful to avoid them during the final days prior to bodybuilding competition. I know of only one or two bodybuilders who will consume milk products right up to the day of a contest.
- Eat your vegetables either raw or as close to raw as possible. It's best to steam vegetables lightly if you must cook them at all. Boiling vegetables in water leaches out most of the vitamins and minerals. Nutritionally, you'd be better off to drink the cooking water than to eat the cooked veggies themselves.
- Always include as much variety in your diet as possible, since this leads to more balanced and healthy eating. Most Americans tend to eat the same ten to twelve foods day in and day out. See if you can build your regular diet to include at least twenty to twenty-five foods, varying them from day to day.
- Eat your food slowly. Eating too quickly often leads to overeating, because the stomach is slow to signal the brain that it has had enough.
- Don't replace food in your normal diet with food supplements. Food supplements are exactly that—supplements to take in addition to the normal diet. Always follow a healthful, well-balanced diet supplemented for nutritional insurance purposes with a sensible amount of vitamins and minerals.
- Try always to consume your supplemental vitamins and minerals with your meals. They will be utilized more efficiently in the presence of other food elements in the digestive tract.
- If you need to gain or lose weight, take a long-term approach to the process. Weight gained quickly is almost 100 percent body fat, while crash dieting eventually leads to binge eating and the ultimate defeat of the diet.

THE PRECONTEST DIET

Ask any bodybuilder about the precontest diet, and she will look at you with a pained expression. That's because the precontest diet is almost always an ordeal, usually a desperate attempt to get down to an abnormally low level of body fat.

Some bodybuilders begin their precontest diet three months before the event; others who are on a very well balanced regular diet don't begin until six weeks or so before the contest. I usually begin my diet about two months beforehand, and I move into it gradually, making it more restrictive as the contest date approaches. By the time I am one month away from the contest, everything is calculated narrowly to bring out the cuts and striations in my musculature. Every calorie gets counted.

The precontest diet particularly stresses fat elimination. It is not necessarily a healthful diet. Most precontest diets are not balanced and do not contain the essential amounts of all nutrients. Bodybuilders usually supplement their food intake with heavy doses of vitamins, minerals, and trace elements to compensate for the imbalance. However, remember that an overabundance of certain nutrient elements does not mean optimal absorption of those if other nutrients that work in complement with those have been removed from the diet.

Many bodybuilders opt for a high-protein–no carbohydrate–low-fat regime with restricted water intake. They often take in as much as 2 to 3 grams of protein per kilogram of body weight each day. Recall how desperately your kidneys need water with such a high protein intake! Unfortunately, they fail to take into account the body's need for carbohydrates as a preferred energy source.

I recommend a high-protein diet with about 1.5 grams of protein per kilogram of body weight. To that I'd add at least 100 grams of carbohydrate to help absorb the protein, together with a minimum 30 to 50 grams of natural vegetable fats and a small amount of animal fat. Rather than avoiding dairy products or red meat, I advise a controlled intake. They do provide you the essential B-12 vitamins that come strictly from animal sources. Calcium and phosphorous, also essential in your diet, are most easily obtained via dairy products.

Eat many small meals rather than a few large meals. Don't skip breakfast and lunch and count on getting everything in just one large meal sometime during the day.

Common food that I eat during the precontest period include tuna fish salad; broiled skinned chicken breast; hard-boiled egg whites (a good snack that is very high in protein, very low in calories); celery and carrots by the pound; a protein drink made with Weider Muscle Builder protein with a dash of Cambridge diet drink powder for flavor; plain yogurt; and oranges, apples, melons, and strawberries. I stay on this relatively restricted diet for three to four weeks. I will allow myself a "day off" after two weeks to "indulge" in some seafood and a little more salad dressing. I do not stay away from bread entirely, as some do. I have a slice or two of whole-grain bread each day. And I drink gallons of pure spring water.

I do keep a careful log of everything I eat during this time. I write down the calorie intake from carbohydrates, protein, and fat in the diet. That reinforces my awareness of what I'm doing. I can monitor total intake to ensure I keep an optimal balance while holding calories down. And writing it all down helps check any temptation to cheat.

The precontest diet can be depressing because it is so restrictive. It is hard to go out with friends, even to enjoy a meal in a health food restaurant, which may use too much mayonnaise in a tuna fish salad or place a tempting bran muffin beside your plate that isn't in your diet. Inevitably, you wind up doing virtually all your eating at home, where you can control every aspect of intake.

I'll generally start my day with a protein drink. I use two scoops of Weider Muscle Builder protein, mixed in a blender with two cups of pure spring water and a scoop of Cambridge diet drink or fresh fruit for flavor. For lunch I will have fruit and tuna fish salad. I may have the salad in a sandwich, but as contest time approaches I usually choose to eat it plain. For the salad I use only white albacore tuna that comes packed in water, which I rinse under running water for a few minutes to take the salt out.

In the afternoon I will have a piece of fruit for a snack. Then dinner will be a large tossed salad or simply some chicken breast and cut up vegetables (peppers, carrots, celery, etc.) As a rule, I don't eat anything after 7:00 P.M.

There are some treats you can enjoy that are healthful and not too fattening. Plain yogurt with granola mixed in is very satisfying. (Three tablespoons of yogurt with one tablespoon granola make about 50 calories.) Raisins and nuts in small amounts provide a good energy boost during the day. Frozen breakfast yogurt makes a good dessert, or take a Cambridge chocolate dessert mix, which is very like a pudding treat when chilled, but minus all those calories.

When it comes to what to drink, bottled spring water or even plain tap water is good. You can squeeze in fresh lemon or lime to give it flavor. Avoid artifically flavored and sweetened diet sodas. They're low in calories but high in sodium content, which contributes to high blood pressure and can cause you to retain water.

Many bodybuilders practice salt restriction for the same reason I recommend avoiding diet sodas. In general, the American diet tends to incorporate too much salt, so cutting down is a good idea. Restricting salt intake altogether may be carrying things to an extreme, since some sodium is necessary in the diet. Also, the iodine added to most table salt contributes to proper functioning of the thyroid gland.

Here are a few tips for managing a precontest diet:

- When eating omelets, cut down on the intake of yolks. I make omelets with one egg yolk whipped together with four egg whites. You can make omelets with spinach, mushrooms, broccoli, or cheese, being careful of course to limit the cheese so that your calorie count doesn't go too high.
- Some fruits are higher in calories than others, so during the precontest weeks go for the lower-calorie choices. Honeydew melon and cantaloupe are especially low in calories. Avocados and mangos, on the other hand, are high in calories.
- When cooking fish or poultry, wrap it in foil to steam-broil in its own juices, grill it on the barbecue with just lemon juice rubbed in to keep if from drying out, or cook it with a minimal amount of purified butter in a nonstick frying pan. These are all better means of preparation than frying or broiling with regular butter or cooking oil in the usual amounts. (Naturally, all the skin and fat should be removed before cooking.)

The precontest diet is just that—a precontest diet. It is not a steady diet to follow as long as you are at all engaged in bodybuilding. It's a relatively unhealthy diet, especially over the long term. Pay attention to details of diet at all times, but don't compromise your health by trying to stay in contest shape on a continual basis. That's an impossible, unreal goal. Instead, adopt a diet that is well balanced and suits your needs for building muscle mass while holding down the buildup of excess body fat.

BODYBUILDING BASICS | 3

The basic weight training and bodybuilding information in this chapter will form the foundation of your lifetime training philosophy. *Do not take your initial workout until you've read through the material here.* You must first develop an understanding of basic terminology and principles involved. You will experience the best results and the least difficulty if you take care from the very beginning to follow the guidelines set out for you here.

TERMINOLOGY

There are several basic terms you should be familiar with before crashing a weight room.

An *exercise* is the type of movement performed to promote muscle growth—for example, a sit-up or bench press. Sometimes an exercise will be referred to as a *movement*.

The *weight* or *poundage* used in an exercise is the actual weight in pounds (or kilograms) of the barbell, dumbbells, or machine resistance used in an excercise.

A repetition (frequently abbreviated to *rep*) is each individual full cycle of an exercise, such as sitting erect and then lowering your body back to the floor in a sit-up movement.

A *set,* in bodybuilding parlance, is a group of repetitions performed in sequence, followed by a *rest interval* and then often another set. Sets of from six to twelve reps are most frequently performed.

A *routine* is the full accumulation of exercise sets done in one day's workout. A routine is frequently presented as a *training program* in a book or magazine or written up as such in a training diary. A routine may also be referred to as a *workout* or day's *training schedule.*

BASIC VERSUS ISOLATION EXERCISES

There are two major classifications of exercises—basic and isolation—and there are uses for both. Basic exercises work the large muscle groups of your body in concert with smaller muscles. You can use very heavy poundages on basic exercises, and they are used most profitably to build a super degree of strength and muscle mass.

In contrast, isolation movements stress single muscle groups or even part of a muscle group. Isolation exercises are generally performed with moderate poundages to etch details into the body's major muscle groups. Isolation exercises are also excellent for building up an injured joint or muscle group.

Here are commonly used basic and isolation exercises for each of the body's major muscle groups:

BODY PART	BASIC EXERCISES	ISOLATION EXERCISES
Thighs	Squats, leg presses, front squats, stiff-legged deadlifts	Leg extensions, leg curls, sissy squats
Trapezius	Upright rowing	Barbell/dumbbell shrugs
Latissimus Dorsi	Barbell/dumbbell bent rows, seated pulley rows, chins, pull-downs	Nautilus pullovers, bent-arm pullovers
Erector Spinae	Deadlifts, stiff-legged deadlifts	Hyperextensions
Pectorals	Barbell/dumbbell incline/flat/decline presses	Incline/flat/decline dumbbell/cable flyes
Deltoids	Barbell/dumbbell presses, presses behind neck, upright rows	Side laterals, bent laterals, front laterals
Triceps	Lying barbell triceps extensions	Pulley push-downs
Biceps	Barbell/dumbbell curls	Dumbbell/barbell/cable concentration curls
Calves	Standing/seated calf raises	One-legged calf raises
Abdominals	Sit-ups, leg raises	Crunches

Bodybuilders use primarily basic exercises in the off-season in an effort to build greater muscle mass. Prior to a competition, they use primarily isolation movements to accentuate muscle mass. Still, an intelligent bodybuilder will do at least one basic exercise with relatively heavy poundages per muscle group in order to retain as much mass as possible while peaking for a competition.

FREE WEIGHTS VERSUS MACHINES

There has been considerable controversy in recent years about the relative efficacy of using free weights (barbells, dumbbells, and related equipment) and exercise machines (Nautilus, Universal Gyms, *et al.*). The arguments for free weights and against machines generally stems from the manufacturers and distributors of free weights, while the manufacturers and distributors of resistance exercise machines argue for their products and against the use of free weights.

Free weights and related equipment are comparatively inexpensive and are therefore widely available. A great variety of exercises can be performed with free weights, often scores of movements for a single muscle group. But in many exercises, free weights don't place direct resistance on a working muscle over its full range of motion. Most exercise machines provide direct and biomechanically balanced stress to the working muscles, and this is very beneficial to bodybuilders and serious weight trainers. However, there are relatively few exercises that can be done on most resistance machines, often as few as two or three movements per machine.

Most women start training on free weights, then eventually incorporate machines into their workouts. Although exercise machines are quite expensive, many gyms now have them available, and gym memberships amortize the cost of these machines so that virtually anyone can afford to use them. The sooner you can begin training with both machines and free weights, the better.

OVERLOAD AND PROGRESSION

The primary object of weight training is to overload a skeletal muscle to induce it to increase in tone, strength, and mass. There is a direct relationship between the weight you use in an exercise and the development of the muscle(s) stressed by that movement, so you should always try to overload a muscle progressively with greater intensity.

There are three ways in which a bodybuilder increases training intensity in an exercise:

1. She performs a greater number of repetitions with a set weight.
2. She lifts a heavier weight for a set number of repetitions.
3. She does an established number of sets and repetitions with a set weight in less elapsed time.

Contest-level bodybuilders often use the third method, which is called *quality training*. However, most women who train with weights use a combination of lifting heavier weights and doing more reps with a set weight as they progressively increase their training intensity.

If you glance ahead to the suggested training programs in Chapter 6, you will notice that a range of repetitions is suggested for each exercise. As an example, you might be asked to do eight to twelve (8–12) reps of barbell bent rows.

Regardless of the suggested repetition range, you can most easily increase training intensity by beginning to do the exercise for the number of reps suggested by the *lower guide number* (in this case, 8). Then, with each subsequent workout, you can add one or two reps to the total you perform, until you reach the *upper guide number* (12). **49**

Once you reach an upper guide number, you should add 5 to 10 pounds to the bar, drop back to the lower guide number for reps, and slowly begin to work your repetitions back to the upper guide number. Continue progressively increasing resistance in this manner on each exercise, and soon you will be handling fairly substantial poundages in all of your movements.

Here is a sample progression chart for one month of doing barbell curls three times per week for one set of eight to twelve repetitions. ("40 × 8" is shorthand for eight repetitions done with 40 pounds.)

	Monday	Wednesday	Friday
Week 1	40 × 8	40 × 10	40 × 11
Week 2	40 × 12	45 × 8	45 × 9
Week 3	45 × 10	45 × 11	45 × 12
Week 4	50 × 8	50 × 9	50 × 10

In most cases, you will be asked to perform more than one set of each exercise in the routines presented in this book. You should reach the upper guide number of *every* set before increasing your training poundage.

Here is an example of how you would increase intensity for three sets of eight to twelve reps in the bench press:

	Monday	Wednesday	Friday
Week 1	50 × 8	50 × 10	50 × 11
	50 × 8	50 × 9	50 × 9
	50 × 8	50 × 8	50 × 9
Week 2	50 × 12	50 × 12	50 × 12
	50 × 11	50 × 12	50 × 12
	50 × 10	50 × 11	50 × 12
Week 3	55 × 9	55 × 11	55 × 11
	55 × 8	55 × 10	55 × 10
	55 × 8	55 × 9	55 × 10
Week 4	55 × 12	55 × 12	60 × 8
	55 × 11	55 × 12	60 × 8
	55 × 10	55 × 12	60 × 8

Occasionally you won't be able to add a new rep to an exercise from one workout to the next. At other times, you will be able to add two or three new repetitions. But as long as you are *trying* to add reps to each workout, you need not worry about not adding one. Your body is subject to natural fluctuations of energy, and that accounts for your ability or inability to add reps to a movement from one workout to the next.

The amount of weight you add to an exercise once you have reached the upper guide number for reps depends on the muscle group(s) being trained and on your relative condition. Most women can add 5 to 10 pounds to movements for large muscle groups such as the thighs, back, and chest, and 2½ to 5 pounds to exercises for smaller body parts.

The number of repetitions you perform of an exercise has a bearing on the muscular development you achieve with that movement. If you do low repetitions (four to six reps), you will primarily develop muscle mass and strength. High reps (fifteen or more) tend to develop local muscle endurance. Medium reps (eight to twelve) seem to develop muscle quality of the type most valuable to a competing bodybuilder.

TRAINING FREQUENCY

Research physiologists have determined that a muscle needs forty-eight to seventy-two hours of rest following a heavy weight workout in order to recuperate fully from the training session and increase in hypertrophy. (Hypertrophy refers to the increase in muscle mass.) Therefore, you must rest at least one full day between workouts for each muscle group.

At the beginning and intermediate levels of weight training and bodybuilding, you should train your entire body each session and work out three nonconsecutive days each week. Most commonly, beginners and intermediates train on Mondays, Wednesdays, and Fridays, which leaves the weekends free for family activities and other recreational pursuits. You can, however, train any three nonconsecutive days each week that are convenient for you.

As you gain experience as a bodybuilder, you can eventually train more frequently than three days per week by splitting your body in halves or thirds and working only a portion of it each session. This training method is called a *split routine,* and it is discussed in detail in Chapter 5. Even though you train more frequently when following a split routine, you will still rest at least forty-eight hours between workouts for each muscle group.

REST INTERVALS

You should rest approximately sixty seconds between sets. If you rest much less than a minute, your muscles and the remainder of your body will be unable to recover adequately from the last set to do justice to the next set you perform. Your pulse rate will drop under 100 beats per minute and your breathing will return to normal after approximately sixty seconds of rest. Then you should begin your next set.

When you are training large muscle groups such as your thighs and back, you will discover that you need up to ninety seconds rest between sets to recover fully. If you rest more than ninety seconds before starting your next set, however, you risk allowing your body to cool down, which makes your muscles and joints more susceptible to injury.

STARTING POUNDAGES

In the first suggested training program at the end of Chapter 6, I have noted starting weights for each exercise as a function of a percentage of your body weight. Most readers   **51** will find these starting poundages to be appropriate, but a few will discover them to be either too heavy or too light.

I have based these starting weights on "average" women, and many of you are far from being average. Therefore, after the first workout you may need to adjust these poundages upward or downward for some or all of your exercises.

A correct starting weight will allow you to comfortably perform the lower guide number of reps in an exercise. If you can easily complete more than this number of repetitions, the poundage you are using is too light. Should it be difficult or impossible to reach the lower guide number of repetitions, the weight is too heavy, and it should be reduced for the next workout.

When you calculate your starting weights, always round *downward* to the nearest multiple of five pounds. As an example, if you weigh 125 pounds and should do an exercise with 30 percent of your body weight, you would use 35 pounds ($125 \times 0.30 = 37.5$, rounded down to 35).

After four to six weeks of training, you will be far more familiar with your relative strength levels than I could ever be, so you should choose your own starting weights for subsequent workouts. For this reason, I have only suggested starting poundages for the initial workout in Chapter 6.

EXERCISE FORM

To get the most out of each exercise, you should use the body form that places maximum stress on the working muscle(s). This involves precisely following the exercise performance guidelines presented in the exercise descriptions given. Move only those parts of the body that are supposed to be moved in an exercise; keep the rest of your body motionless. Using extraneous body motion to "cheat" up a weight should be strictly avoided.

You must also move a barbell or other weight *slowly along the full range of motion allowed by the joints that are bent and straightened* during the execution of an exercise. Doing partial movements gives your working muscles only partial benefit.

Quick, jerky movements can be avoided by raising and lowering a weight relatively slowly. As a rule of thumb, take two or two and one-half seconds to raise a weight upward and three or six seconds to lower it back to the starting point. You should always attempt to lower a weight a bit more slowly than you raised it, because there is a natural tendency to drop a weight from the top of a movement back to the starting point. Dropping a weight lessens the value received from an exercise and increases the chance of injuring yourself.

BREATHING PATTERNS

I have noticed considerable confusion about how to breathe while training with weights. Some experts suggest breathing in upon exertion and out during the relaxation phase of a movement; others suggest exhaling upon exertion and inhaling during the relaxation phase; and still others suggest letting nature decide when you inhale and exhale during an exercise.

After careful investigation, I have concluded that it is best to exhale as you lift a weight and inhale as you lower it. *Never* hold your breath while training with weights. Holding your breath while exerting yourself can build up enough pressure within the chest to impede the flow of oxygenated blood to and from your brain, causing you to faint. It also causes dangerously high but momentary elevations of arterial blood pressure. Scientists call this effect a *Valsalva maneuver,* and it can be disastrous if it occurs when you are doing bench presses or other movements performed with a heavy weight while lying on your back.

BREAK-IN AND MUSCLE SORENESS

In most cases, weight training will stress your muscles much more intensely than any other form of physical activity that your have undertaken. As a result, training with weights can cause your muscles to become very sore if you don't gradually break in to maximum-intensity training.

Referring to the beginning-level training schedule outlined at the end of Chapter 6, you should begin your gradual break-in to heavy training by doing only one set of each listed exercise for the first week that you work out. For the next week, you can do two sets of each exercise for which multiple sets are listed, and beginning with the third week you can perform the entire program.

You should avoid straining with the weights during your break-in cycle, because it will take three or four weeks of steady training before your muscles are in sufficiently good condition to train with maximum intensity. Until then, I recommend that you terminate each set one or two repetitions before you would reach the point where you must struggle to complete a rep.

Each time you switch from one training program to another, you should also work out with less intensity for the first two or three sessions. Your muscles won't be accustomed to handling the unique stresses provided by new exercises until you have put in a couple of workouts at less than normal intensity.

Even if you break into a new training program slowly and carefully, you may experience mild muscle soreness. Frequent warm and soothing baths are the best way to alleviate muscle soreness.

RECORD KEEPING

One of the best ways to make sense of how each exercise, workout, and training technique affects your body is to use a training diary. Ordinarily, you won't be able to see changes in your physique, strength levels, or general fitness level from day to day or even from week to week. But by recording your workouts and periodically reviewing your records, you can easily identify the effects that a variety of external training and dietary stimuli have on your body.

You can use any notebook or ledger book to keep a training diary, or you can purchase one of several commercially produced training diaries available at bookstores. Most of the diaries I have seen used by champion bodybuilders have had bound pages rather than spiral bindings.

At a minimum, you should record the date of each workout, the exercises you do, the weights of each exercise, and the sets and reps performed. You can use a variation of the weight training shorthand briefly presented in the section on resistance progression earlier in this chapter.

If you do a barbell curl for three sets of ten reps with 40 pounds, it would look like this when recorded in bodybuilding shorthand: *barbell curl: 40 × 10 × 10 × 10.*

A series of sets of squats in which you did eight reps for two sets and only seven for a third would look like this: *squat: 75 × 8 × 8 × 7.*

And, four sets of bench presses in which you increased the weight and decreased the reps with each succeeding set might look like this: *bench presses: 50 × 12, 60 × 10, 70 × 8, 80 × 6.*

Using this shorthand, you can easily record an entire workout in compact form. And you can refer back to recorded data many years later and still instantly understand what you recorded.

Other data that you can record each day in your diary include your body weight, the time you start and finish each workout, the day of the week, your relative energy level and mood each workout, how much and how well you slept the night before, how your workout went, and any other factors that would have an effect on how well your workouts go each day.

You might also record what you eat every day, as well as the time of day you eat each type of food. Don't forget to include your food supplements and the actual amount of each food that you consume.

Once you have a few weeks of data included in your diary, don't let it just sit there. Schedule regular times to review your diary. Try to identify periods during which you made especially fast gains, and to identify what caused these improvement spurts. In the end, you will find your training diary a much more reliable record of progress than your memory.

SAFETY RULES

Weight training is a relatively safe form of exercise that can be made almost totally safe by following these twelve safety rules:

1. Never train alone. Since there are normally groups of women and men working out at health spas and gyms, this rule doesn't apply to these structured situations. In a home gym it is often difficult to work out with someone present to act as a safety spotter. Try to cultivate a training partner from your family or neighborhood acquaintances. Or have a nontraining friend or family member present while you are working out.

While you might have a personality that makes it better for you to train alone, most body builders and serious weight trainers prefer to work out with a training partner. As you become more experienced at weight training, the intensity of your workouts must inevitably be increased, and you will need a training partner to assist you with forced reps, negative reps, descending sets, and other intensified training techniques.

It will prove valuable to develop a sense of camaraderie with your training partner, each of you verbally driving the other to push harder to complete a difficult rep or two.

You will also find it more difficult to miss a workout when you know that your training partner is patiently waiting for you down at the gym.

2. Use a spotter. This is an outgrowth of Rule 1—having a spotter is a primary reason for not working out alone. A safety spotter should stand alertly in position to catch the bar in case you can't complete a repetition of bench presses or squats. You won't normally need a safety spotter when performing exercises with dumbbells or machines.

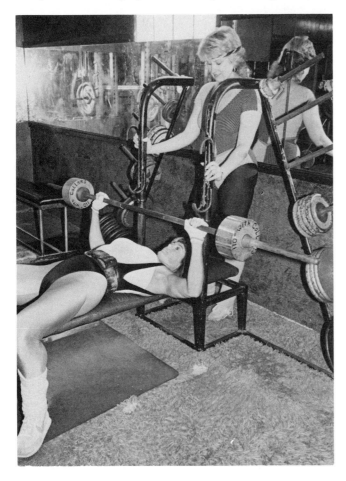

Here Terry Doyle, both a gym owner and my coach's daughter, acts as my spotter on bench presses.

3. Use catch racks. Many pressing benches and squat stands have special catch racks set at a lower level than the normal rack, and you can place a barbell there when you are unable to complete a squat or bench press rep. Always use these catch racks when they are available.

4. Don't lift a barbell that doesn't have its collars firmly set. If you extend your arms or legs unevenly when using a barbell without collars, the weights will slide off one end, causing the weighted end to whip violently downward, probably resulting in an injury.

5. Wear a weight-lifting belt. The heavier you train—and particularly if you have incurred any injury in prior sports participation—the more important it becomes for you to use a weight-lifting belt and/or body wraps. These protective devices can keep you from either injuring or reinjuring yourself pumping heavy iron.

Weight-lifting belts are made from thick, tough leather. They are either four or six in-   **55**

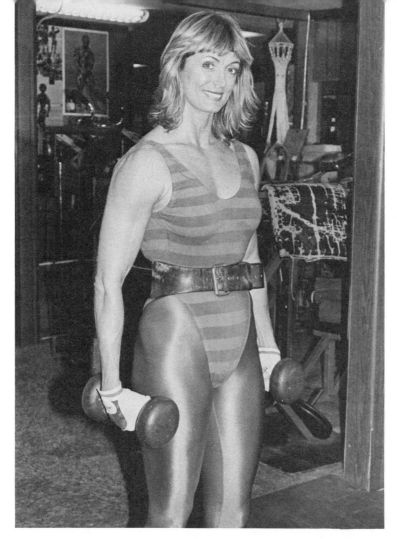

ches in width across the back. The four-inch belt is used in competition; the six-inch belt can be used only in training. Since the six-inch belt provides greater protection to the lower back and abdomen, you should purchase the wider belt. (Weight-lifting belts can be purchased at many sporting goods stores or through advertisements in weight training and bodybuilding magazines. They range in price from about $25 to more than $50 for a custom-made belt.)

Always use a weight-lifting belt to protect your lower back and abdomen when doing squats, heavy back exercises (barbell bent rows, deadlifts, etc.), and overhead lifts (military presses, dumbbell presses, etc.). Cinch the belt tightly around your waist for each set and loosen it immediately following the set.

You can also use joint wraps to support a joint or muscle and to keep an injured joint or muscle warm while training. Elastic gauze wraps are those most frequently used for support. They should be wrapped moderately tightly in one or more layers over an injured area. If you are wrapping an injured joint, it's best to use a criss-cross pattern as you wrap the joint.

In recent years neoprene rubber bands have also been used to keep an injured joint or muscle group warm during a workout, thereby reducing the chance of reinjury. For maximum support and protection, you can use both fabric and neoprene rubber wraps. I know a woman bodybuilder with a history of knee injuries who is able to do very heavy squats using both types of wraps. First she slips the neoprene bands over her knees, then dons warmup pants. Finally, she wraps her knees over the warmup pants with gauze wraps. Using this wrapping system, she can comfortably use heavy weights in her leg

exercises.

6. Warm up thoroughly before training. Most minor weight training injuries could be prevented if all bodybuilders warmed up prior to a weight workout. The proper way to warm up will be discussed in detail in the next chapter.

7. Don't train in an overcrowded gym. Resting too long between sets while waiting for a piece of equipment will allow your body to cool down, an open invitation to injury.

8. Never hold your breath. As discussed earlier in this chapter, holding your breath can cause you to pass out.

9. Train under competent supervision. This rule is particularly applicable to women in their first few weeks of training, since an experienced woman or man watching you work out a couple of times can help you avoid minor training errors that might eventually lead to injuries.

10. Maintain good gym housekeeping. Keep all loose plates off the floor, and return barbells and dumbbells to the proper racks as soon as you are finished using them. Equipment lying at random on a gym floor will eventually trip someone.

11. Use proper biomechanical positions on all exercises. Poor body form when doing exercises magnifies the chance of injury while performing movements. Adhere to the instructions provided in the exercise descriptions in this book, and you will obviate this injury risk.

12. Obtain all possible information about weight training and bodybuilding. The more informed you are about all facets of training with weights, the less likely it becomes that you will be injured.

RECUPERATION

Your muscles require two or three days of rest in which to recuperate from a workout and increase in hypertrophy. And in general, your body needs adequate sleep and rest to promote full recuperation.

Individual sleep requirements vary widely. I'm sure we all know individuals who require as little as four or five hours of sleep each night. Thomas Edison, the great inventor, slept only one or two hours per day throughout his most productive years, taking occasional catnaps during the day. He certainly lost none of his mental acuity in the process. At the other end of the scale, many individuals appear to require ten or more hours of sleep each day to avoid being zombies all day.

Most authorities consider eight hours to be the optimum length of time for sleep each night, primarily because of the old axiom that the day should be divided into thirds—eight hours of work, eight hours of personal pursuits, and eight hours for sleep. You will probably function best on seven to eight hours of sleep each day. As long as you awake fully rested each morning, you have allowed yourself sufficient sleep.

In order to be sure you sleep and rest enough, be careful to avoid late night study and recreational hours, which can result in a whole day spent yawning and trying to concentrate. Don't be afraid to take a short nap in the afternoon if you find yourself dragging late in the day. An afternoon siesta is institutionalized in many societies.

WATCH WHAT YOU EAT

All bodybuilders and most other individuals who train with weights for physical fitness or improved athletic performance carefully monitor their diets, because improvements from weight training can be seen more quickly and dramatically when a woman follows a healthy diet. Indeed, most women bodybuilders feel that diet is up to 50 percent of the battle, particularly in the weeks just prior to a competition. Refer to Chapter 2 for the guidelines to follow.

You can also add to your knowledge of nutrition by reading books and magazine articles on the subject. The nutrition articles in *Muscle & Fitness* and other weight-training and bodybuilding magazines provide an excellent starting point for building your knowledge of sports nutrition.

MENTAL CONCENTRATION

There are two mental techniques that you can use to improve the quality of your workouts—concentration and visualization. If you intend to be a successful competitive bodybuilder, you *must* master these two mental techniques. Training and nutrition are important to a bodybuilder, but they can't get the job done if the mind doesn't potentiate the chance for success.

You can develop markedly greater muscle mass and functional strength by consciously flexing a working muscle as strongly as possible under resistance and then fully and forcefully extending it. It's only possible to achieve this type of powerful muscle contraction and extension through pinpoint concentration on the working muscles.

In order to develop unbreakable concentration, you must first understand exactly which muscles are being stressed by each exercise. You can determine the primary muscle group being stressed in each exercise by reading the "Exercise Emphasis" section for each movement in the workout chapters. Also, review the illustrations of muscle anatomy presented in Chapter 1.

Once you fully understand the muscle group on which you should concentrate during an exercise, focus your mental energies on it throughout each set. Imagine it contracting and extending with each repetition. Feel it getting larger as it pumps full of blood. Feel it beginning to burn as fatigue wastes build up. Initially you may find it easier to visualize the muscle working by standing in front of a mirror and actually watching it contract and extend under heavy resistance.

At first you won't be able to focus your mind on a working muscle for more than a few seconds at a time. If you keep practicing this concentration technique, however, you will begin to improve the length of time you can concentrate. Ultimately you will be so deeply into the working muscle group during a set that a truck could crash into the side of the gym without your noticing it until after your set.

Visualization also provides a practical means of programming your subconscious mind to help you succeed in reaching long-term goals. Once you have properly programmed your subconscious mind, you will find it easy to avoid missing workouts and to avoid eating foods that hold back your progress. It will be easier as well to conform to every other facet of a disciplined bodybuilding lifestyle.

This use of visualization takes advantage of a psychological construct called *self-actualization*. Essentially, self-actualization involves thinking you can do something long enough and hard enough so your subconscious mind brings you to the point where you can actually do it. Have you ever seen a girl who was so sure she would be a singer when she grew up that she actually became one? Or a physician? Attorney? Champion athlete? These are examples of self-actualization in action.

To use visualization to good advantage, you must first set goals for yourself to reach. Make these realistic goals that you can reach within a few months. Once you set a realistic goal, spend ten to fifteen minutes each day visualizing yourself reaching that goal. As a bodybuilder, I try to visualize every muscle as it will appear on my physique at my next competition, almost as though my mind is projecting a three-dimensional image of my physique just behind my eyelids. I actually get to the point where I can feel my body the way it will soon become.

I've found it best to practice this kind of visualization at a time of the day during which I will be relaxed and free from distractions, such as just before falling asleep each night. And I put in my visualization practice each day to assure myself of programming my subconscious mind sufficiently to guarantee success.

Programmed like this, your subconscious mind begins automatically to make those choices that lead you painlessly to success in weight training and bodybuilding. (Visualization also works quite well in all other arenas of life. Give it a try!)

DEVELOPING A TRAINING INSTINCT

Every successful athlete learns to listen to the biofeedback his or her body provides and to react to this information with subtle shifts of training philosophy. To a bodybuilder, developing this "training instinct" is of paramount importance, because it ultimately allows you to determine the relative value of the complete spectrum of exercises, routines, and training techniques you follow. Only by experimenting with each training variable and evaluating it with your training instinct can you concentrate your efforts primarily on those factors that yield maximum results.

It takes approximately a year of observing biofeedback signals to develop a true feel for how well a particular training variable works on your body. But once developed, this instinct for bodybuilding training and diet will help you to chart an infallible course to bodybuilding success.

So, how should you go about developing a flawless instinctive training ability? First you must learn to look for and appreciate the biofeedback signals your body gives you. Have you ever run as hard as you can until you had to stop and catch your breath? In such a case, your heavy breathing was a biofeedback signal telling you you'd pushed too hard and had to eliminate an oxygen debt before continuing.

In bodybuilding, the ultimate biofeedback signal is the appearance of your physique. If it is gradually improving, you know you are on the right track. Unfortunately, however, a woman bodybuilder's physique improves so slowly and imperceptibly that muscle growth isn't a very good biofeedback signal to monitor.

Most bodybuilders seek a muscle "pump"—the tight, blood-congested feeling in a muscle that signals that a muscle has been optimally trained. A good pump is a pleasant feeling and a good indication that you have trained hard enough to induce muscle hypertrophy.

The following are other biofeedback signals monitored by champion bodybuilders and what each should tell you about your body:

- Persistent and chronic fatigue—you are probably overtraining or undersleeping.
- Muscle soreness—you have trained a muscle either significantly harder than normally or from a new angle.
- Increased appetite—as long as it is an appetite for healthful, muscle-building foods, this is a good indication that you are entering a period of very fast muscle growth.
- A burning sensation in a muscle during a workout—you are pushing that muscle very close to the point of total collapse. This burning sensation is called the "pain zone," and all top bodybuilders seek it.
- A quick and noticeable increase in body fat—your diet is too high in calories.
- An increase in exercise poundages—your muscles are growing larger. (There is a direct correspondence between the amount of weight you use in an exercise and the mass of the muscles that move the weight.)

By consistently monitoring these and other biofeedback signals, you will soon develop good instinctive training ability. Once you have developed this ability, you will be able to tell within only two or three workouts if a particular exercise, routine, or training technique is of value in your overall training regimen.

REFINING YOUR PROGRAM | 4

Once you've mastered the basics and actually been training with weights for a number of weeks, you are ready to start introducing refinements into your program. In fact, that's a virtual necessity. Each individual responds uniquely to all the training variables, so you can only make the best gains for you by learning how to formulate your own training program.

To begin with, concentrate on sharpening your training instinct. You must have well-developed instincts in order to formulate optimum individualized routines; you have to learn what works best for your body. For example, you may have been doing incline presses with a barbell and/or two dumbbells for months with only a small increase in upper pectoral development. When you try incline presses on a machine, your upper chest almost explodes into new growth. Obviously that tells you to include the machine variation of incline presses in your routines.

At more advanced levels of training, you will probably find you make your best gains when following a split routine, which I'll introduce you to in a moment. And when formulating your own training schedules, be sure to plan in maximum intensity and a minimum number of sets in order to avoid overtraining. I do not recommend performing more than six to ten total sets for large body parts (e.g., thighs, back, and chest) or more than four to six sets for smaller muscle groups.

In any program, it's best to train torso muscle groups before your arms in workout, because your weaker arm muscles already limit the degee to which you can stress your larger and more powerful torso groups. Fatiguing your biceps and triceps by training them before your back, chest, and shoulder muscles only worsens this situation. (I'll discuss how to make your arms effectively stronger than your torso muscle groups in discussing pre-exhaustion techniques later in this chapter.)

SPLIT ROUTINES

Each time you hit the gym for a workout, you have only a finite amount of energy to expend on that workout. That amount of energy will slowly increase with hard and steady training and a good bodybuilding diet, but it is still limited.

Eventually your workouts will be long and/or hard enough that you exhaust your energy reserves before you can train your entire body in one workout. This is when you should begin using a *split routine,* dividing your body into halves or thirds and training only part of it each workout day.

Even when using a split routine, you must have at least forty-eight to seventy-two hours of rest between workouts for each muscle group in order to allow for full recuperation and growth. A muscle can be resting while another part of your body is working, so you can train for muscle growth in one area even as the muscles in another area are recuperating from a previous day's workout.

The simplest form of split routine—and the one you should use most of the time—involves splitting your muscle groups into two equal portions, training one half on Mondays and Thursdays and the other half on Tuesdays and Fridays. Many bodybuilders find this four-day split routine ideal for off-season mass-building, because it allows ample time between workouts for each muscle group to recuperate.

The most common division of body parts for a four-day split routine involves working those muscles that push against the weights one day and those that pull the next day. Here is a typical "push-pull" division of body parts:

Monday/Thursday	**Tuesday/Friday**
Abdominals	Abdominals
Chest	Thighs
Shoulders	Back
Triceps	Biceps
Forearms	Forearms
Calves	Calves

Another typical division of body parts for four-day split routine training involves a scheme of training the torso one day and the limbs the next:

Monday/Thursday	**Tuesday/Friday**
Abdominals	Abdominals
Chest	Thighs
Shoulders	Upper Arms
Back	Forearms
Calves	Calves

You will notice that abdominals, calves, and forearms are stressed in each workout in the foregoing programs. All three of these muscle groups can profitably be trained as often as five or six days per week. You will discover that abdominal training done first in your weight workout serves as a very good full-body warm-up.

Another step up the ladder of training intensity is a five-day split routine in which you work out each of the five weekdays and take the weekend off training. Typically, you will divide your body into halves as for a four-day split, working the first half on Monday, Wednesday, and Friday and the second half on Tuesday and Thursday the first week.

Then, during the second week, you do the half that was trained only twice the previous week on Monday, Wednesday, and Friday.

Designating the Monday/Thursday split of either four-day program as "A" and the Tuesday/Friday split as "B", here is how one month of five-day split routine training would look.

	Monday	**Tuesday**	**Wednesday**	**Thursday**	**Friday**
Week 1	A	B	A	B	A
Week 2	B	A	B	A	B
Week 3	A	B	A	B	A
Week 4	B	A	B	A	B

There are two forms of six-day split routines, both of which add even greater intensity to a workout. In the first of these six-day splits, you train each major muscle group twice per week, dividing your body into thirds.

Here is an example of how you can divide your major muscle groups into thirds for a six-day split routine:

Monday/Thursday	**Tuesday/Friday**	**Wednesday/Saturday**
Abdominals	Abdominals	Abdominals
Chest	Shoulders	Thighs
Upper Back	Upper Arms	Lower Back
Calves	Forearms	Calves

The foregoing six-day split routine is excellent for use during the final four to six weeks of precontest training, when you are attempting to add overall hardness to your physique. In a few rare cases, competitive bodybuilders react well to this six-day split during an off-season cycle. For most bodybuilders, however, off-season six-day-per-week workouts quickly result in an overtrained state.

A minority of bodybuilders can profit from using a six-day split routine in which major muscle groups are trained three days per week during the precontest cycles. In such a six-day split you must divide your body parts into halves as for the four-day and five-day split routines. Then train one half on Mondays, Wednesdays, and Fridays, the other half on Tuesdays, Thursdays, and Saturdays. Most bodybuilders would quickly burn out on this type of six-day split routine, however.

CHANGING ROUTINES

The object of bodybuilding training is to place a progressively greater overload on a muscle group to keep it gaining in hypertrophy. Unfortunately, the human body and mind are so adaptable that they frequently require more than merely a progressive increase in training intensity to continue improving mass, strength, and muscle tone.

After several weeks of steady training on a set routine, your body will usually adapt to that routine and cease to continue improving its hypertrophy. Then you should change to a new training program in order to force your body to adapt to a new regimen.

While a majority of bodybuilders with stoic personalities can keep making gains on a particular training program seemingly *ad infinitum*, I suggest that you change to a new routine each four to six weeks. A few bodybuilders I've known over the years physically and mentally adapt to a new program so quickly that they need to change to a new routine virtually every workout.

Ultimately, you can experiment with training for different lengths of time on a set schedule in order to determine what works best for you. For now, however, follow each suggested routine in this book for four to six weeks before switching to a new program.

MUSCLE CONFUSION   Bodybuilders vary widely in physical and mental temperament. There are stolid, plodding women who never become bored with a set training program and continue with it for years at a time. On the opposite side of the coin, there are women who quickly become bored with a training program and quickly stop making gains if forced to stay on the same program for an extended period of time. And, of course, there are women who fall at points between these two extremes.

For women who quickly become bored with a set training program, I recommend use of the muscle confusion technique. This involves never doing the same training program twice in a row. From day to day, you vary the exercises used, the sets, the reps, the training tempo, and even the training principles themselves in your workouts. In essence, you use a non-routine routine for your training.

A non-routine routine keeps the muscles off balance, confused about what they will be hit with next. As a result, they can't settle into a comfortable groove; they are forced to continue increasing in hypertrophy to handle each unfamiliar new stress.

At the same time, your mind is constantly stimulated by new challenges when you follow a non-routine routine. The net effect is continued good bodybuilding gains, because both mind and body are stimulated by the new and unique stresses that you devise to test yourself in the gym.

POWER WORKOUTS

Many women wish to increase their strength levels. At first I trained for added power to improve my rebound ability as a basketball player. Later I wanted to increase basic body strength—particularly in my shoulder, arm, and forearm muscles—so I could handle the relatively heavy work involved in orthopedic surgery.

There are many reasons why you might wish to improve your physical power. Regardless of why you wish to increase your strength levels, any power improvement goal can be achieved with basically the same workout. You must train with heavy weights and low reps on exercises that stimulate primarily the larger muscle groups of your body.

In order to train safely with low reps (i.e., one to five reps for power building), you must first do a few lighter, higher-rep sets of an exercise to warm up your working muscles and joints thoroughly. The best way to combine high-rep warm-up sets with low-rep strength-building sets is to pyramid your reps and training poundages. This involves starting an exercise with a light weight for high reps, then progressively adding weight and decreasing reps on each succeeding set.

Here is a typical weight-rep pyramid for the squat:

Set Number	Reps	Weight
1	12	100
2	10	135
3	8	155
4	6	170
5	4	185
6	2	200

On occasion you can do a single repetition to accelerate the strength-building pyramid further, but you should do maximum singles no more than once every two weeks. Performance of max singles too frequently will quickly burn you out. You can also do a final "pump set" of twelve to fifteen reps with a greatly reduced weight if you have enough available energy. Many bodybuilders are enthusiastic about the results they receive from such a pump set.

The following is a good strength-building split routine that you can use to rapidly build strength.

MONDAY/THURSDAY

Exercise	Sets	Reps
1. Incline sit-ups	3	15–20
2. Hyperextensions	3	10–15
3. Squats*	6	12,10,8,6,4,2
4. Stiff-legged deadlifts*	3	10,8,6
5. Barbell bent rowing*	5	12,10,8,6,4
6. Barbell shrugs*	4	12,10,8,6
7. Barbell curls*	4	10,8,6,4
8. Barbell wrist curls *	4	12,10,8,6
9. Seated calf raises*	5	15,12,10,8,6

TUESDAY/FRIDAY

Exercise	Sets	Reps
1. Hanging leg raises	3	10–15
2. Incline barbell presses*	6	12,10,8,6,4,2
3. Nautilus pullovers*	5	10,8,6,4,2
4. Military presses*	5	10,8,6,4,2
5. Lying barbell triceps extensions*	4	10,8,6,4
6. Barbell reverse curls*	4	10,8,6,4
7. Dumbbell wrist curls*	4	12,10,8,6
8. Standing calf raises*	5	15,12,10,8,6

NOTE: Exercises marked with an asterisk must have reps and weights pyramided.

At first glance this might seem too abbreviated a routine. But when training with very heavy weights to increase your strength, you will find your body unable to handle more than this amount of work. Indeed, if you added too many sets to this suggested program, you would soon become overtrained. (Please see the caution on overtraining at the end of this chapter.)

TRAINING THROUGH MUSCLE FAILURE

Training through muscle failure is one of two approaches used by champion bodybuilders to stimulate muscles to more rapid development. (The other approach is use of supersets.)

To understand how to train past the point of momentary muscle failure, you must first understand what it means to train *to* failure. Training to failure involves continuing a set until you literally can't complete a full repetition under your own power. As an example, you might continue a set of strict barbell curls until your eight repetition stalls out only a third of the way to the top of the movement.

THE CHEATING PRINCIPLE

If you can force a muscle to keep working as hard as possible *past* the point at which it normally fails, you will thereby work it harder than is normally possible and will stimulate much greater gains in hypertrophy. The simplest way to push a muscle past the normal failure point is to use the cheating principle, which involves using muscles other than the ones being stressed in a movement to assist you in completing a repetition that you might normally not have finished on your own.

Beginning bodybuilders are always cautioned against cheating. They are told to use good, strict form in all of their exercises in order to stress all of their muscle groups maximally. For a beginner, this is good advice, because novice bodybuilders invariably use cheating form to remove stress from a muscle group. You will use it to place more stress on the muscle.

To correctly use the cheating principle, you must *first do a set of a movement to failure in strict form.* Then when you do fail, you can use extraneous muscle groups to impart just enough impetus to the bar to boost it past the point at which it has failed to pass on its upward path. Finally, you lower the bar on your own while resisting its downward momentum with all of your power.

Let's use barbell curls to illustrate correct use of the cheating principle, and let's assume that you have loaded up the bar with 70 pounds and failed to complete the eighth rep. After you have failed, swing your torso backward and forward just enough to allow you to pull the bar up to your shoulders in a cheating movement. Lower it back to the starting point and do another cheating rep.

There's a limit to how many cheating reps at the end of a set are of value to a bodybuilder. In my experience, you need do no more than two or three. Past three reps, your working muscles will have become so completely fatigued that no amount of additional work will be beneficial.

FORCED REPS

Cheating reps can be performed training alone, as long as you don't use them for dangerous movements like bench presses. If you have a training partner, however, you will probably make better use of forced reps to push your muscles well past the failure point.

Forced reps allow for more precise removal of just the right amount of weight to allow completion of a repetition past failure, because your training partner pulls up on the middle of the bar just enough to remove that weight. When you're relying on cheating to "remove" weight, you can never be as precise about how much is actually "taken off."

As with cheating, you begin forced reps by pushing a set to the point of normal muscular failure. Let's say that you're doing bench presses with a heavy barbell and your training partner standing at the head end of the bench to assist you. Failure means that you

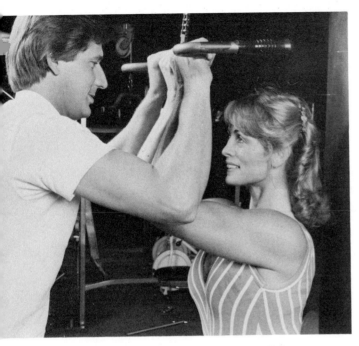

An example of forced reps on Nautilus pull-downs.

Forced rep on Nautilus leg extension machine.

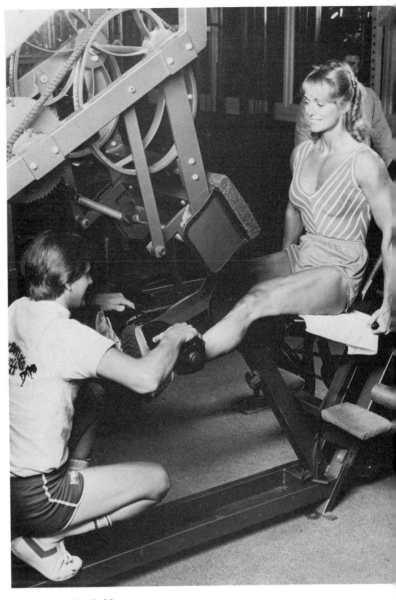

can't complete a final rep with the amount of weight on the barbell. However, you can no doubt complete the rep with a bit less weight.

So, once you fail with a repetition, your partner pulls up on the bar to remove 5 pounds—perhaps a little more—allowing you to complete a forced rep. Then he or she pulls up a bit harder for a second forced rep (since your muscles are growing more and more fatigued) and perhaps even harder for a third forced rep. As with cheating, you won't get much benefit from going more than two or three forced reps.

SUPERSETS

Another good way of increasing training intensity is to reduce the average amount of rest between sets, and one of the best ways to do this is to perform supersets. Supersets are groupings of two exercises—either for antagonistic muscle groups or for the same muscle group— performed with an absolute minimum of rest between sets and a rest interval of normal length between supersets.

The least intense form of superset is done for antagonistic muscle groups, such as the biceps and triceps. Here are examples of typical supersets for a variety of antagonistic muscle groups:

biceps+triceps=barbell curls+pulley push-downs
biceps+triceps=preacher curls+lying triceps extensions
pectorals+lats=bench presses+lat machine pull-downs
pectorals+lats=parallel bar dips+seated pulley rows
quadriceps+hamstrings=leg extensions+leg curls

A more intense form of superset involves performing a compound of two exercises for a single muscle group. Here are some common examples of supersets done for a single body part:

chest=incline presses+cable crossovers
trapezius=upright rowing+shrugs
lats=chins+pullovers
biceps=preacher curls+standing barbell curls
triceps=dumbbell triceps extensions+pulley push-downs
deltoids=side laterals+bent laterals
quads=squats+leg extensions

A specialized form of superset for a single muscle group makes use of the training technique called pre-exhaustion.

PRE-EXHAUSTION

If you look at an anatomy chart, you can easily see that the biceps and triceps muscles of the upper arms are smaller than the deltoid, trapezius, latissimus dorsi, and pectoral muscles of the torso. And the arm muscles are not only smaller, but also *weaker* than the torso muscle groups.

Unfortunately, your arm muscles work in concert with those of your torso when you do basic exercises for your pecs, traps, delts, and lats. For example, when you do bench presses for your chest and front deltoid muscles, your triceps also get into the act. And the unfortunate factor in this is that the smaller arm muscles tire and fail to move the weight long before the larger and stronger torso muscles have been stressed to the max.

Because your torso muscles are so much stronger than your biceps and triceps, it's impossible for you to stress your chest, shoulder, and back muscles sufficiently through normal training procedures to promote optimum hypertrophy in them. However, by using the technique of pre-exhaustion you can briefly make your arms as strong as your torso muscles. More accurately, you can temporarily weaken your torso groups to make them as weak as your biceps and triceps.

Pre-exhaustion involves supersetting an isolation movement for a torso muscle group with a basic exercise for the same body part. As an example, you can work your pectorals with dumbbell flyes and bench presses. The flyes willl pre-exhaust your pecs, making them briefly much weaker than usual. If you then immediately begin a set of bench presses with a barbell, you can take advantage of this brief weak state of your pecs to use your momentarily stronger arms to push your pecs very hard.

68   It's essential that no more than five seconds rest be allowed between exercises in a pre-

exhaustion superset, because the pre-exhausted muscle recuperates and regains its initial strength very quickly. Within ten to fifteen seconds, it will be more than 50 percent recovered to its original state. Therefore, you must plan your superset so you have the equipment for each exercise in the superset immediately at hand. Otherwise, you will end up resting the pre-exhausted torso muscle group excessively just in the walk across the gym for the second movement of the superset.

Here are typical pre-exhaustion supersets for each torso muscle group:

    upper pecs = incline flyes + incline presses
    lower pecs = decline flyes + decline presses
    pecs (in general) = flyes + bench presses
    deltoids = side laterals + presses behind neck
    traps = shrugs + upright rows
    lats = pullovers + lat machine pull-downs

You can also do a triset (three consecutive exercises with no rest between movements) to pre-exhaust your thighs to a maximum degree before doing squats. In this case, your pre-exhaustion triset will consist of leg presses, leg extensions, and squats.

All bodybuilders who train with the intent of placing maximum stress on the working muscles in the shortest possible length of time use pre-exhaustion supersets and trisets. And they work wonders in pushing the torso and thigh muscles to the max.

A CAUTION ON OVERTRAINING

I haven't mentioned overtraining earlier, because you won't have built up the volume of training at the beginning level that results in an overtrained state. Overtraining results when your workouts become so long that your body can't fully recuperate between them. Overtraining results only from workouts that are too long, not from training sessions that are too intense.

There is a dynamic energy balance in your body that is much like a checking account. You are constantly withdrawing energy via your workouts, much as you deplete a checking account by writing checks. And you are constantly depositing energy through rest and the maintenance of a good diet, just as you make periodic deposits in your checking account.

If you use up more energy than you deposit, you can go "energy broke," overtrain. It's like overdrawing your checking account. When you go energy broke, the bank won't hassle you, but your body rebels by becoming ill or otherwise refusing to accept any more lengthy workouts.

Here are the seven most common symptoms of an overtraining:

   1. Lethargy
   2. Lack of appetite
   3. Illness
   4. Persistently sore muscles and/or joints
   5. Lack of enthusiasm for training
   6. Insomnia
   7. Elevated morning pulse rate

If you experience one or more of these symptoms, you are beginning to overtrain. To combat overtraining, begin by taking a one-week layoff from weight workouts. Actually, you can normally prevent overtraining simply by taking a one-week layoff every three or four months.

At the end of your layoff, get back into the gym, but be sure that you initiate your weight workouts with a totally new training program. Your new routine should have at least 20 percent fewer total sets than the last one you used, and your training intensity should be at least 20 percent greater than in the past. This procedure will solve your overtraining problem and make it less likely you will overtrain in the future.

WARM-UPS AND SUPPLEMENTARY EXERCISES | 5

While it is not essential that you take a warm-up prior to training with weights, warming up thoroughly will improve the quality, effectiveness, and safety of a body-building workout. Researchers have concluded that a good warm-up prior to strenuous exercise fulfills the following vital functions:

- It readies muscles and joints to accept heavy stress and makes the muscles and joints more flexible, greatly reducing the chances of injury.
- It improves neuro-muscular coordination, reducing the chance of moving a weight out of its normal, safe biomechanical groove, thereby lessening the chances of injury.
- It reduces muscle and connective tissue viscosity, allowing you to lift significantly heavier weights than if you hadn't warmed up.
- It prepares you mentally to drive strongly through a heavy workout.

An ideal preworkout warm-up consists of five to ten minutes of light aerobic exercise, stretching movements, and calisthenics, followed by one or two light, high-rep sets of a basic exercise for each major muscle group just before it is trained. At the end of your warm-up, you will probably be perspiring lightly, your pulse rate will be moderately elevated, and you will be physically and mentally ready for a stiff workout.

Many warm-up patterns have been suggested, but I have had best success using this sequence of exercise. (Descriptions of each follow.)

1. Jogging in place or jumping rope—two to three minutes
2. Alternate toe touches—twenty to thirty reps
3. Front torso stretch—thirty to sixty seconds
4. Jumping jacks—twenty to thirty reps
5. Push-ups—ten to twenty reps
6. Standing hamstring stretch—thirty to sixty seconds for each side
7. Sit-ups—twenty to thirty reps
8. Wall calf stretch—thirty to sixty seconds with each leg
9. Torso twists—thirty to fifty reps

71

10. Thigh stretch—thirty to sixty seconds with each leg
11. Freehand squats—twenty to thirty reps
12. Shoulder (towel dislocate) stretch—eight to ten stretches

If you proceed through this routine with a minimum of rest between exercises, it should take you no more than ten minutes to complete your nonweight warm-up. Follow it with one or two light, high-rep sets of a basic exercise for the major muscle group to be worked first, and you'll be prepared to tackle maximum training poundages safely and aggressively.

WARM-UP EXERCISE DESCRIPTIONS

JOGGING IN PLACE/ JUMPING ROPE — Both of these light forms of aerobic exercise will be familiar to everyone. The key to performing either of these types of exercise correctly in a warm-up is to begin with a slow cadence and low knee lift with each step. Then slowly accelerate the cadence of your steps or skips, raising your knees higher and higher until you are jogging or jumping at a fast pace at the end of your two or three minutes of activity.

ALTERNATE TOE TOUCHES — Stand with your feet spread about three feet apart and keep your legs straight throughout the movement. Extend your arms directly out to the sides (parallel to the floor) and keep your arms straight throughout the movement. Bend forward and twist to the left to touch your left foot with your right hand. Return to the starting position and repeat the movement to the right side. Alternate sides until you have done the suggested number of repetitions to each side.

FRONT TORSO STRETCH — Lie facedown on the floor and stiffen your body. Straighten your arms so you are supported only on your toes and hands, as in the starting position for a push-up. Keeping your arms and legs straight, lower your hips as close as possible to the floor, if not actually to the floor, and throw your head back. Hold this stretched position for at least thirty seconds.

PUSH-UPS — Assume the same starting position as for torso stretching. Bend your arms and lower your chest down to touch the floor. Push yourself back to the starting point and repeat the movement. If you find it difficult to do push-ups in this position, you can make the movement somewhat easier to perform by resting your knees rather than your toes on the floor.

STANDING HAMSTRING STRETCH — Stand erect with your feet about six inches apart and stiffen your legs. Slowly bend forward at the waist as far as comfortably possible. Grasp your calves or ankles to gently assist in pulling your torso as close as comfortably possible to a position against on your thighs. Hold the stretched position for at least five to six seconds, then relax.

SIT-UPS — Lie on your back and hook your toes beneath a restraining bar or heavy piece of furniture. Bend your legs at 30-degree angles to remove stress from your lower back, and keep them bent throughout the movement. Fold your arms across your chest. Lift your head and shoulders from the floor and slowly curl your torso from the floor, lifting first your upper back and then your lower back until your torso is perpendicular to the floor. Return to the starting point and repeat the movement.

Stand facing a wall, about three feet back from the wall. Lean forward, place your hands on the wall a bit below shoulder level, and stiffen your body. Slowly force your heels toward the floor to stretch your calf muscles. If you can easily place your heels on the floor, walk backward a few more inches and try the movement again. Hold the stretched position for the suggested length of time, five to six seconds, then relax your calves. *WALL CALF STRETCH*

Stand in the same starting position as for alternate toe touches. Keeping your arms at shoulder level, twist your torso as far to the left as possible, allowing your left arm to travel to the rear and your right arm to cross your chest. Twist back as far as you can in the other direction and continue twisting back and forth until you have done the suggested number or reps to each side. *TORSO TWISTS*

Stand facing a solid object on which you can place your left hand to balance your body as you do the stretch. Bend your right leg fully and grasp your right foot behind your buttocks with your right hand. Pull gently upward on your right foot to stretch your right thigh muscles. Hold the stretched position for at least five to six seconds. Be sure to stretch your left thigh for an equal length of time. *THIGH STRETCHES*

Stand with your feet set at about shoulder width, your toes angled slightly outward. Extend your arms directly forward (parallel to the floor) and leave them in this position throughout the movement to assist body balance. Keeping your torso as upright as possible and your heels on the floor, slowly bend your knees and lower your body down into a full squatting position. Return to the starting point and repeat the movement for the desired number of repetitions. *FREEHAND SQUATS*

Stand erect with your feet set at about shoulder width. Grasp the ends of a towel and straighten your arms downward so the towel rests across your upper thighs. Keeping your arms straight, slowly raise your hands in a semicircular arc up over your head, then backward and downward until the towel rests across the backs of your upper thighs. At a position somewhat behind your head, you will feel a kinetic stretch in your shoulders and chest muscles. Return your hands to the starting point of the movement and repeat it for the suggested number of repetitions. *SHOULDER (TOWEL DISLOCATE) STRETCH*

STRETCHING ROUTINES

As a bodybuilder, you will find stretching an excellent supplement to your weight workouts. Stretching allows you to achieve a longer range of motion in all of your

73

bodybuilding exercises, and this longer range of motion results in a better quality of development. My experience is that you can expect an improvement of up to 10 percent in physique if you include stretch flexibility in your overall training and fitness program.

I've already described a couple of stretching exercises good as warm-ups before getting into weight workouts. There are additional benefits from stretching. As well as generally contributing to overall health and physical fitness, it improves athletic ability and relieves tension. By its action on the muscles and at the joints, it promotes flexibility and thereby reduces the risk of injury to either from trauma or overextension. Because of the benefits, you may want to adopt stretching as part of your daily fitness routines.

HOW TO STRETCH

Most women either stretch too hard or bounce forcefully into a stretched position, thereby losing much of the value of the exercise. To stretch correctly, you must do it gently. Unless you stretch slowly and gently, you will receive very little benefit from a program of stretching exercises.

Two specialized forms of neurons (nerve endings) within your muscles will dictate how you stretch.

The first type acts as a stretch-reflex mechanism to protect your muscles and joints from being suddenly stretched so far that a muscle tears or a tendon ruptures.

To illustrate how the stretch-reflex mechanism protects you, imagine yourself running down a mountain trail in the dark. Your toes unexpectedly come down on a rock and the heel of your foot suddenly drops below the level of your toes. Without the stretch-reflex mechanism, your calf muscle would be stretched so fast and far that it would be torn. However, when the stretch-reflex neurons in your calf sense that the stretch is progressing too quickly, they stimulate a reflexive contraction in your calf. This contraction acts as a shock absorber to slow and then stop the stretch before your calf is injured.

The stretch-reflex mechanism can be triggered by any quick and forceful stretch, including a stretching exercise into which you throw yourself. The stretch reflex automatically *shortens* a muscle, and that prevents you from achieving a full stretch. That's why a bouncing stretch is counterproductive.

A second type of neuron within your muscles senses when a stretch has progressed too far, sending a pain signal to tell your brain that you shouldn't stretch any farther. If you stretch into this pain zone too far, you will in fact tear enough tiny muscle fibers to make your muscles quite sore for several days.

Stretching into the pain zone yields less of an improvement in flexibility than stretching to a point just short of the pain zone and holding that position. You can begin by holding a stretch for five seconds, then gradually work the duration up to half a minute. More than a minute per stretch produces diminishing returns. To stretch a muscle or joint optimally, you should ease slowly into position, taking about thirty seconds to get fully stretched. This slow entry into a stretch effectively circumvents the stretch-reflex mechanism, allowing you to achieve a deep stretch comfortably.

As you move into a stretched position, approach the pain edge, then back off just enough so you feel no discomfort in the stretched position. Hold this position for an appropriate length of time. In many ways this method of achieving and holding a stretch is identical to that used by Yoga advocates. (Yoga also yields good results in flexibility improvement.)

Don't expect an overnight increase in flexibility, because that is a very slow quality to develop, much slower than strength or aerobic endurance. It takes persistence and near-daily stretching exercise sessions to slowly improve body flexibility.

74

Here are several widely used stretches you can employ in addition to those described as warm-ups in a personal stretching exercise program.

Emphasis. This exercise stretches all of the muscles of the thighs and hips, particularly the hamstrings.

Hurdler's Stretch

Starting position. Sit on the floor with your left leg extended directly forward and held straight throughout the stretch. Bend your right leg fully and place the inside of it flat against the floor. Distribute your weight equally between the two legs.

Stretched position. Lean forward over your left leg to stretch your hamstring muscles. If you have sufficient flexibility, you can grasp your left ankle to pull your torso forward over your left leg. Be sure to do an equal amount of stretching with your right leg in the forward position.

Emphasis. This exercise stretches the hamstrings, the muscles of the inner thighs, and the lower back muscles.

Seated Hamstrings Stretch

Starting position. Sit on the floor and spread your legs as wide as possible. Keep your legs straight throughout the stretch.

Stretched position. Bend forward and bring your torso as close to the floor as comfortably possible.

Emphasis. The lunging stretch stretches the frontal thigh muscles, buttocks, and hamstrings.

Lunging Stretch

Starting position. Stand erect with your feet set a comfortable distance apart and your hands on your hips. Step forward two and a half to three feet with your left foot. Keep your right leg nearly straight throughout.

Stretched position. Slowly bend your left leg as fully as possible and bring your hips as close to the floor as you comfortably can. Be sure to do an equal amount of stretching with your right foot in the forward position.

Emphasis. This exercise stretches all of the muscles on the insides of your thighs.

Inner Thigh Stretch

Starting position. Sit on the floor with your legs bent and the soles of your feet against each other. Pull your feet as close to your hips as possible.

Stretched position. Push down on your knees to stretch the inner thigh muscles.

Emphasis. All movements in which you bend to the side stress the muscles on the sides of the torso, particularly the oblique muscles at the sides of the waist.

Side Bend Stretch

Starting position. Stand erect with your feet set a little wider than your shoulders. Extend your arms and clasp your hands directly above your head. Maintain this arm position throughout the stretch and keep your legs straight.

Stretched position. Bend directly to the right as far as comfortably possible. When you finish bending to the right, bend back to the left for an equal length of time.

Emphasis. This exercise stretches primarily the pectoral muscles of the chest. Secondary stress is placed on the shoulder muscles.

Chest Stretch

Starting position. Stand with your back to a countertop, horizontal bar, or high table. Extend your arms to the rear and place your palms flat on that stationary object. Keep your arms straight throughout the stretch.

Stretched position. Keeping your hips directly beneath your shoulder joints, slowly bend your legs to create a stretched sensation in your chest and shoulder muscles.

75

Doorway Stretch

Emphasis. Using this stretch, you can stretch the muscles of your chest and shoulders more intensely than with the shoulder (towel dislocate) stretch.

Starting position. Stand in a doorway and place the palms of your hands against the insides of the doorjamb about six inches above the level of your hip girdle. Lean a little forward and fully straighten your arms.

Stretched position. Slowly lean far enough forward to stretch the muscles of your chest and shoulders fully.

Neck Stretch

Emphasis. This exercise acts on the muscles at the front, back, and sides of your neck.

Starting position. Stand erect with your feet set a comfortable distance apart and your hands on your hips.

Stretched position. Incline your head as far directly forward as comfortably possible and hold this stretched position for an appropriate length of time. Next stretch the muscles on the front of your neck by inclining your head backward. Finish by inclining your head both to the right and to the left.

Hand/Wrist Stretches

Emphasis. This flexibility exercise stretches all of your fingers, your hands, and your wrists.

Starting position. Stand erect with your feet a comfortable distance apart. Raise one hand to a position a bit above waist level and grasp the thumb of it with your other hand.

Stretched position. Slowly bend your thumb backward until it reaches the stretching zone. Continue by stretching every finger in this manner. Finally, interlace your fingers with your palms facing away from your body, and force your elbows toward each other to stretch your entire wrist-hand structure.

A SUGGESTED STRETCHING PROGRAM

As mentioned earlier, you will obtain optimum results from a flexibility-training program if you perform it on a near-daily basis. The best options are to use stretching either as part of your warm-up or as a beneficial cool-down session following a workout. I personally prefer a post-workout flexibility-training session to stretching at any other time of the day.

Here is a sample stretching program that you can use either as presented or adapt to your own unique needs:

Stretching Exercise	Minimum Duration (sec.)	Maximum Duration (sec.)
1. Standing hamstring stretch	5	30
2. Wall calf stretch	5	30
3. Hurdler's stretch	5	30
4. Front torso stretch	5	30
5. Lunging stretch	5	30
6. Front thigh stretch	5	30
7. Inner thigh stretch	5	30
8. Side bend stretch	5	30
9. Towel dislocate stretch	5	30
10. Doorway stretch	5	30
11. Neck stretch	5	30
12. Hand/wrist stretches	5	30

You can vary the order of these stretches if you like. Begin by doing five seconds in each stretch, gradually working up to thirty seconds per stretch. I suggest that you add five seconds per week to a stretch, until you are up to the full thirty seconds. Finally, be certain that you do the same amount of stretching for each side of your body on all one-armed and one-legged stretches.

AEROBICS

If you're aiming for optimum physical fitness, you must give emphasis to all three forms of exercise—weight training, stretching, and aerobic exercise. All physical conditioning experts firmly believe that a person must possess high levels of strength, flexibility, and cardio-respiratory (heart-lung) endurance to be truly physically fit.

The word *aerobic* is derived from the Greek word meaning *with oxygen*. Aerobic exercise is long-lasting physical effort carried on at a low enough intensity so the body can supply oxygen to the working muscles at least as fast as it is burned up. The most familiar forms of aerobic activity include running, walking, cycling, swimming, and participating in dance or exercise classes.

Physiologists have determined that a woman must exercise to accelerate her pulse rate to above 130 beats per minute and maintain it at that level for at least fifteen minutes to achieve an aerobic effect (i.e., to improve the condition of her lungs, heart, and circulatory system). During aerobic exercise, you can occasionally monitor your pulse rate by placing the fingers of one hand just above your collarbone, where your neck merges with your torso. Simply count the heartbeats in six seconds and add a zero to that figure for your working heart rate.

You can easily gauge whether or not you are exercising aerobically by doing it with another person. You should be running (or doing any other form of aerobic exercise) slowly enough so you can carry on a conversation with your training partner.

You will also hear or read about *anaerobic exercise,* or exercise *without oxygen.* Anaerobic exercise is of such high intensity that it uses up oxygen much faster than the body can supply it, resulting in an oxygen debt. This oxygen debt quickly becomes so great that you must stop exercising. Sprinting on a track, in the pool, and on a bicycle are each forms of anaerobic exercise.

I am drawing the distinction between aerobic and anaerobic exercise, because it has a bearing on how you metabolize body fat when you are attempting to lose weight. Anaerobic exercise burns primarily the glycogen (sugar) stored in your muscles and liver and results in a minimum loss of fat. In contrast, aerobic exercise burns fat quite efficiently, both during a workout and for several hours afterward, since aerobic exercise elevates the body's basal metabolic rate.

In order to give you an accurate idea of how much fat can be burned through aerobic exercise, here is a chart of the number of calories burned in thirty minutes of continuous activity in seven popular forms of exercise:

Activity	Calories
Running (10 mph)	450
Bicycling (15 mph)	350
Swimming (1 mph)	325
Racquetball	250
Tennis	200
Basketball	150
Walking (3 mph)	100

Keep in mind that you will also continue burning calories at a somewhat accelerated rate for hours after an aerobic workout. For the sake of reference, you must expend 3500 calories more than you eat to burn off one pound of body fat.

Competitive bodybuilders, who must briefly reach a very low body fat percentage for contests, make extensive use of aerobic exercise prior to a championship. I personally run and ride a bicycle for one or two hours per day during a competitive cycle. And, it's not unusual to hear of a woman bodybuilder who has ridden a stationary bicycle through three one-hour television shows each evening for several weeks prior to a competition!

I have found that it is counterproductive to schedule aerobic exercise either just before or just after a weight workout. It is much better for you to schedule an aerobic session at least four hours before or after your bodybuilding workout. Close to a competition, a woman bodybuilder experiencing difficulty stripping away every ounce of body fat may even find it a good practice to do an aerobic workout twice per day. She can bicycle in the morning, pump iron during the middle of the day, and run at night.

ADVANTAGES AND DISADVANTAGES

Aerobic exercise improves endurance, increases energy, prevents heart and vascular degeneration, burns body fat, relieves tension, tones the body, improves local muscle endurance, and promotes a youthful appearance. Some researchers have even concluded that there is a relationship between aerobic exercise and longevity.

On the negative side of the coin, aerobic exercise doesn't improve strength or muscle mass to anything near the degree provided by weight training. And running actually decreases flexibility. Most distance runners are very inflexible athletes with particularly tight hamstrings.

Many endurance athletes also develop overuse injuries such as tendinitis, shin splints, persistently sore muscles, and bursitis. You can usually avoid these injuries by switching daily from one form of aerobic exercise to another. If you do feel an injury developing, you don't need to be compulsive about continuing your aerobic program on a daily basis. Take a day or two off aerobic training. Rest does wonders for overuse injuries.

POPULAR AEROBIC ACTIVITIES

The safest form of aerobic exercise is swimming, provided you *can* swim. All of the body's weight is buoyed by the water as you swim, so there is very little stress on the joints. So if you have a pool or other suitable body of water available, make swimming a part of your aerobic training program.

Cycling allows you to support much of your body weight on the bicycle seat, so it also places little harmful strain on your joints. There is, however, a small chance that you will be involved in an cycle crash and injured. Cycling is an excellent activity for building cardio-respiratory endurance. If you fear open-road cycling, ride a stationary bike. Bicycle racers and cross-country skiers consistently test out with the best levels of cardio-respiratory endurance.

Running is by far the most popular form of exercise (estimates of participation range form 10 percent to 15 percent of the American population), but it presents a greater injury potential than either swimming or cycling. Each foot comes crashing down on the pavement thousands of times during a training run. As a result, runners suffer numerous injuries to their lower extremities, particularly to their feet, ankles, shins, and knees. Breaking slowly and sensibly into a program of regular running, then running only three or four days per week, will allow you to avoid most running injuries. You can profitably fill non-running days with bicycling and swimming workouts.

Exercise and dance studios everywhere offer aerobic exercise classes, which can also help you burn off excess calories. While these classes build only a limited degree of muscle tone and very little solid muscle tissues, they *do* allow you to burn calories in an enjoyable manner. Depending on the intensity of an aerobic exercise class, you can burn off 150 to 250 calories in a one-hour session.

CHEST EXPANSION

Since your rib cage consists of bones and not muscles, it would seem unlikely that you could increase the volume of your chest. But, it can be done and should be done if you wish to develop maximum upper body impressiveness.

Chest expansion is accomplished by combining a deep breathing exercise with a chest stretching movement. This technique slowly stretches the cartilages that connect your ribs to your sternum (breastbone). This lengthens your ribs and expands your chest structure.

It is easiest to increase the volume of your rib cage if you are still in your teen years, because the rib cartilages are most pliable and more easily stretched at that age. Later in life, the cartilages harden, and it becomes more difficult to stretch them. In either case, however, rib cage expansion is a very slow process that demands a great deal of persistence and patience.

The movement that you perform to prompt chest expansion is the breathing squat. This exercise is merely a regular full-range squat performed with a set number of deep breaths between each movement. Since you are trying to expand your rib cage and not the girth of your thighs, you should use a relatively light weight when performing breathing squats. Something in the range of 50 percent to 75 percent of your body weight is appropriate. (You may want to refer to the description of conventional squats—given on page 82 of this book—to help develop your understanding of the movements involved.)

Once you have the weight across your shoulders and have set your feet in the proper position for squats, take three very deep breaths, exhaling and then inhaling as fully as possible on each breath. Hold the third breath while you squat down and return to the starting position. Exhale and repeat the process for ten repetitions. Then for the next ten reps, take four breaths between each repetition, and for a final five reps you should take five breaths each time. This gives you a total of twenty five repetitions of breathing squats, which should leave you somewhat breathless.

As soon as you place the barbell back on a squat rack, immediately lie down and do twenty five repetitions of breathing pullovers. This is merely a stiff-arm pullover (see page 161) movement performed with a barbell or a single dumbbell held in both hands. Breathe in as deeply as you can on the downward cycle of the movement, and hold your breath until you return the weight to the starting point.

LEVEL ONE WORKOUTS 6

Now that all of the preliminaries are behind us, I am sure that you are eager to actually begin working out. In this chapter I will describe twenty-three resistance exercises for all areas of your body. Then I will outline three progressively more difficult workouts that you can use for the next three to four months. As soon as you have read this chapter, you can don your training ensemble and give the first of these three workouts your best shot.

While I describe twenty-three exercises in this chapter, there are enough permutations of each movement to actually give you seventy-five to one hundred "exercises" for use in future workouts. Several of these movements can be done on two or three types of equipment, each of which affects the working muscles a bit differently. Many other movements can be performed using a variety of grip widths and foot placements, each of which also attacks your muscles from a slightly different angle.

Regardless of how long you continue to train with weights, you will periodically repeat most of these exercises in your workouts. Therefore, it's essential that you learn to perform each movement correctly from your first workout. Read each exercise description, carefully reviewing the start and finish positions depicted for the movement, and you should be able quickly to master the exercise without additional coaching.

Until you have firmly established the neuromuscular coordination necessary to execute each exercise smoothly—a process that shouldn't require more than three or four workouts—it will feel somewhat clumsy to perform the movements. This is perfectly normal. Within a few workouts, however, you will have learned to do the exercise so well that you will no longer need to think about how to perform it—you will have mastered the exercise.

You will systematically master more and more bodybuilding exercises until you eventually have at your command literally hundreds of movements from which to choose when formulating your own advanced workouts. Many additional exercises will be presented in the chapters that follow. You will learn even more new bodybuilding movements through further reading and by observing others training in your gym.

Give each new exercise that you encounter a four- to six-week trial in your workouts, carefully observing its effect on your working muscles. Certain exercises have a much greater positive effect on a muscle group than others, and those should most frequently be included in your workouts. A few movements will prove to be worthless. However, you will not discover which exercises have the best effect on your unique body without testing every available bodybuilding movement.

THIGH AND HIP EXERCISES

SQUATS
Exercise Emphasis

Bodybuilders consider squats to be the best exercise for developing the muscles of the thighs (particularly the quadriceps), buttocks, and hips. Secondary emphasis is placed on the abdominal muscles and the erector spinae muscles of the lower back. Squats are also a valuable exercise for athletes. Researchers have concluded that the fastest runners invariably have superior quadriceps strength.

Starting Position

Place a barbell on a squat rack set at a height four to six inches lower than the level of your shoulders, and load the bar to an appropriate weight for a set of squats. Duck under the bar, bend your legs about 30 degrees, place your feet directly beneath the bar, and position the bar across your shoulders at the base of your neck behind your head. Balance the bar in this position throughout the movement by grasping it about halfway between your shoulders and the barbell plates on each side. Straighten your legs to remove the barbell from the rack, and step backward enough to be free of the rack. If the bar presses painfully into the skin over the vertebrae of your neck when held in this position, pad the middle of the bar by wrapping a towel around it. Place your feet shoulder-width apart and angle your toes slightly outward. Tense your back muscles to keep your torso upright throughout the movement. Focus your eyes at a point on the wall in front of yourself at head level, and maintain this focal point throughout the movement.

Movement Performance

Keeping your torso erect, slowly bend your knees and sink into a full squatting position. As your legs bend, your knees should travel a few inches forward and slightly outward, directly over the toes of each foot. Without bouncing at the bottom of the movement, slowly straighten your legs to return to the starting point of the exercise. Repeat the movement for the required number of repetitions.

Exercise Variations

If you have poor ankle flexibility, you will find it impossible to do squats with your feet flat on the floor. Every time you attempt to bend your legs fully, your heels will automatically rise from the floor, resulting in a precariously balanced bottom position of the squat. You can effectively neutralize this problem by squatting with heels elevated. Place your heels on either a two-by-four-inch board or two thick barbell plates as you squat, and ankle inflexibility will no longer be a problem.

Advanced bodybuilders frequently perform partial squats. You can do parallel squats (bending your legs only until your thighs are parallel to the floor), half squats (squatting only halfway down to the full squatting position), and quarter squats. You can also do bench squats in which you straddle a flat exercise bench and squat down until your buttocks lightly touch the surface of the bench. On each of these partial movements, you will be able to use a heavier weight than for a normal full squat.

Many bodybuilders have found it valuable occasionally to vary their foot position for squats. Doing squats with a wider stance stresses the inner thigh muscles more intensely, while squatting with a narrow foot placement shifts stress more to the midthigh muscles.

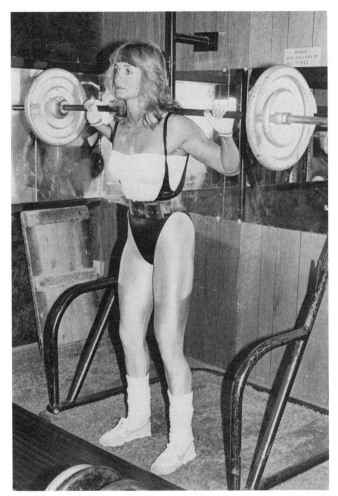 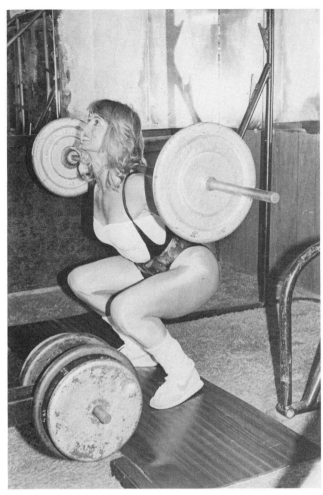

Start.   **Finish.**

Angling your toes more acutely outward will stress the muscles on the lower and inner sections of your thighs. Angling your toes slightly inward places greater stress on the lower and outer sections of your thighs.

Lunges are an excellent movement for stressing the quadriceps, buttocks, and hamstrings, but with less intensity than is provided by squats. Generally speaking, bodybuilders perform squats to increase thigh muscle mass and lunges to improve the shape of their thighs and buttocks.

LUNGES
Exercise Emphasis

Place a barbell weighing approximately 30 percent as much as used for squats behind your neck in the same position as for a set of squats. Stand with your feet set eight to ten inches apart and your toes pointed directly forward. You won't need a board under your heels for balance when doing lunges.

Starting Position

Keeping your torso erect throughout the movement, step forward approximately three feet with your left foot. With your right leg held relatively straight, slowly bend your left leg as fully as possible. At the bottom position of the movement, your left knee should be several inches ahead of your left ankle and your right knee will be four to six inches above the floor. In this position, you will feel stress in the buttock and hamstring muscles

Movement Performance

83

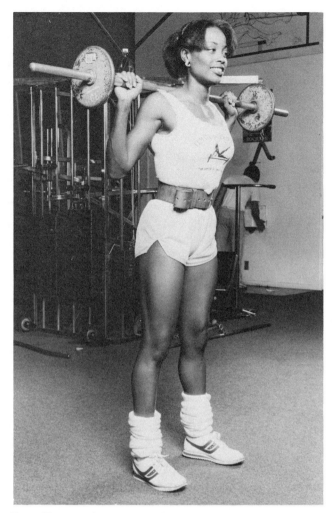 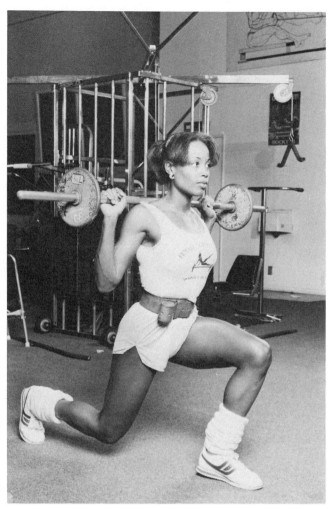

Patsy Chapman demonstrates the starting position. . . . and the finish.

of your left leg and in the quadriceps of your right leg. Slowly straighten your left leg and push yourself back to the starting position. Do the next repetition with your right foot forward. Alternate forward feet until you have done the desired number of repetitions with each leg in the forward position.

Exercise Variations

If you have been physically inactive and your legs are weak, you should initially do lunges *without* added resistance. Simply place your hands on your hips when doing the movement. Should you have any difficulty with your balance when using a barbell, you can easily solve the problem by holding two light dumbbells down at your sides instead as you do the movement. Holding dumbbells, you can move your hands a bit from side to side to maintain balance.

LEG EXTENSIONS
Exercise Emphasis

Leg extensions isolate resistance directly on the quadriceps muscles. Very little stress is placed on any other muscle group.

Free-Weight Starting
Position

Sit on the padded surface of the machine with your legs toward the movement arm of the apparatus. Slide forward until the backs of your knees are at the edge of the machine's padded surface. Hook your insteps under the lower set of roller pads (if there are two sets). Sit erect and grasp the edges of the seat pad to steady your body in position during the movement.

Sit in the Nautilus leg extension machine in the same position as on a free-weight machine. With the Nautilus machine, however, you can lean back against an angled back support and grasp a pair of handles at the sides of your hips to steady your body in position during the movement. Many Nautilus leg extension machines have an adjustable back support that can be moved either toward the lever arm of the machine for women with shorter thigh bones or away from the movement arm for long-legged women. If the back support is adjustable, it should be positioned so the backs of your knees are at the edge of the seat pad when you are lying back against the support. A movable handle beside your right hip can be lifted to remove teeth from a gear behind the seat while the back support is repositioned. Simply lower the handle to lock the back support in position for your set of leg extensions.

Nautilus Starting Position

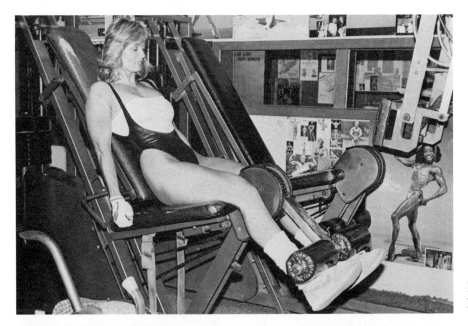

Beginning movement on the Nautilus leg extension machine.

Legs at full extension

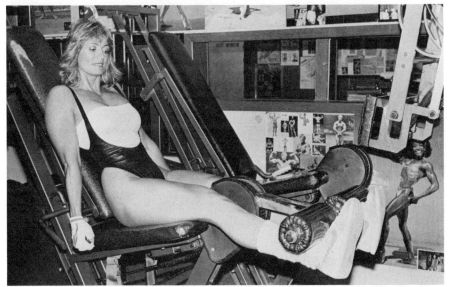

Universal Gyms Starting Position This position is the same as on a free-weight leg extension machine.

Movement Performance Slowly extend your legs under resistance until they are locked in a straight position. Hold this position for a moment before lowering the weight back to the starting point of the exercise. Repeat the movement for an appropriate number of repetitions.

Exercise Variations You can do this exercise with one leg at a time, a practice that allows you to use greater mental concentration on each repetition. When you can focus all of your mental energies on one working arm or leg, rather than splitting your attention between two limbs, you achieve a significantly more intense contraction in your working muscles. This principle of mental concentration applies to all exercises in which you use one arm or leg at a time.

LEG CURLS Exercise Emphasis Leg curls isolate resistance directly on the biceps femoris muscles at the backs of your thighs. Minor secondary stress is placed on the muscles of the calves.

Free-Weight Starting Position Lie facedown on the padded surface of the leg curl machine, with your feet toward the movement arm of the apparatus. Slide your body toward your feet until your knees are near the edge of the pad. Hook your heels under the upper set of roller pads (if there are two sets). Straighten your legs fully and grasp the edges of the padded surface to steady your body in position during the movement.

Nautilus Starting Position Assume the same position as for leg curls on a free-weight machine. The only difference is that the Nautilus machine has handles to grasp near the head end of the bench.

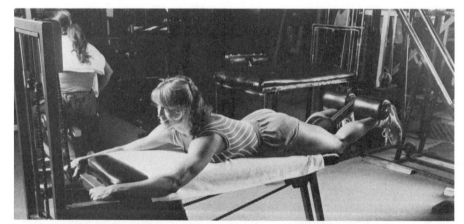

Beginning movement on the leg curl machine.

Finish.

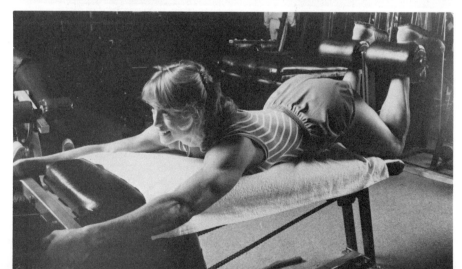

This is the same starting position as on a free-weight leg curl machine. *Universal Gyms Starting Position*

Being careful to keep your hips in contact with the padded surface of the machine, use the strength of your hamstring muscles to bend your legs as fully as possible. Hold this fully bent position for a moment, then let the weight slowly straighten your legs. Repeat the movement for the required number of repetitions. Don't let your hips rise from the pad, as that markedly shortens the range of motion over which your hamstrings contract and extend. *Movement Performance*

As with leg extensions, you can perform leg curls one leg at a time. In recent years, a leg curl machine has been developed that allows a bodybuilder to do the movement one leg at a time while in a standing position. *Exercise Variations*

CHEST EXERCISES

Bench presses strongly stress the pectorals, deltoids, and triceps. Minor secondary stress is placed on the latissimus dorsi. *BENCH PRESSES Exercise Emphasis*

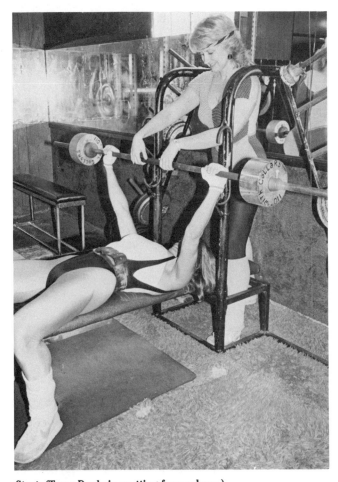
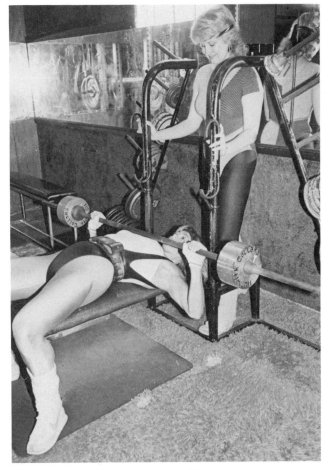

Start. (Terry Doyle is spotting for me here.)   Finish.   87

Free-Weight *Starting Position*	Place a barbell on the rack of a pressing bench and load it to an appropriate poundage. Lie back on the bench with your head toward the rack, and place your feet flat on the floor on either side of the bench. With your palms toward your feet, grasp the bar with your hands set four or five inches wider than your shoulders on each side. Straighten your arms to take the weight off the rack, and balance the barbell directly above your shoulder joints.
Nautilus Starting *Position*	Adjust the Nautilus double chest machine seat as high as it will go. Sit in the seat and fasten the seat belt over your lap. Place your feet on the movable platform in front of your legs and push against the platform enough to bring the pressing handles forward where you can grasp them with your palms toward each other. With another push of your feet to assist your pressing muscles, straighten your arms.
Universal Gyms *Starting Position*	Lie on the bench with your shoulder joints directly beneath the handles of the pressing lever arm. Place your feet in a comfortable position on the floor on either side of the bench. With your palms toward your feet, grasp the middle of the pressing handles. Straighten your arms fully.
Movement Performance	Being careful that your upper arm bones travel directly out to the sides at 90-degree angles to your torso, slowly lower the barbell down to touch the middle of your chest lightly (or, in the case of Nautilus and Universal machines, lower the handles as far past the level of your chest as possible). Press the bar or handles back upward until your arms are straight. Repeat the movement for the required number of repetitions.
Exercise Variations	When using a barbell for bench presses, the main exercise variation involves changing grip width. To a lesser entent, this variation also applies to bench presses on a Universal Gyms machine. Doing benches with a relatively wide grip tends to place maximum stress on the front portion of the deltoids and the outer edges of the pectorals. Bench presses performed with a narrow grip shifts major stress to the triceps and the inner sections of the pectorals.
INCLINE PRESS *Exercise Emphasis*	Incline presses are merely bench presses done lying on an angled bench rather than on a flat pressing bench. All chest exercises performed on an incline bench stress the upper portions of the pectorals, the front portion of the deltoids, and the triceps.
Starting Position	Load a bar resting on the rack of an incline bench to an appropriate poundage for a set of incline presses. Lie back on the bench. (Some incline benches have a seat on which you can sit, while others have two angled foot rests on which you can stand.) Take the same grip on the barbell as you would for a bench press, and straighten your arms to remove the barbell from the rack. Support the barbell at straight arm's length directly above your shoulder joints. When viewed from the side, your arms will appear to be perpendicular to the floor.
Movement Performance	Being sure to keep your elbows back, slowly lower the barbell down to touch the upper part of your chest lightly. Press the weight back to straight arm's length. Repeat the movement for the desired number of repetitions.
Exercise Variations	The same grip-width variations used for bench presses can be used when doing inclines, although a narrow grip is seldom used for incline presses. You can also change the angle

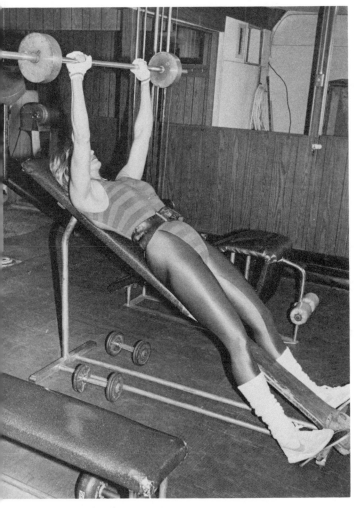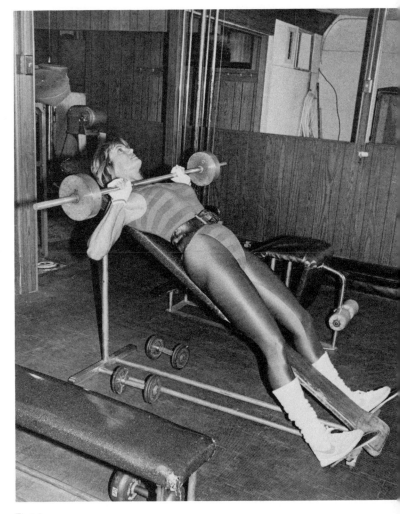

Bench set at 45-degree angle. Start.   **Finish.**

of some incline benches, which results in a slightly different type of stress being placed on the upper chest, deltoid, and triceps muscles. Most commonly, incline benches are set at a 45-degree angle. If your bench angle is adjustable, try a 30-degree angle for a few sets of inclines. Actually, any angle from 5 degrees above parallel with the floor to almost 90 degrees can be successfully used when doing incline presses.

Flyes isolate resistance primarily on the pectoral muscles. Secondary stress is placed on the front part of the deltoids. Unlike with bench presses, there is little or no triceps involvement when doing flyes.

FLAT-BENCH FLYES
Exercise Emphasis

Grasp two light dumbbells and lie back on a flat exercise bench. Place your feet flat on the floor on either side of the bench. Extend your arms directly above your shoulder joints, your palms toward each other. Bend your arms slightly and keep them bent throughout the movement. Press the dumbbells lightly together directly above the chest.

Starting Position

Slowly lower the dumbbells directly out to the sides in semicircular arcs to as low a position as comfortably possible. At the bottom position of the movement, you should feel a stretch-

Movement Performance

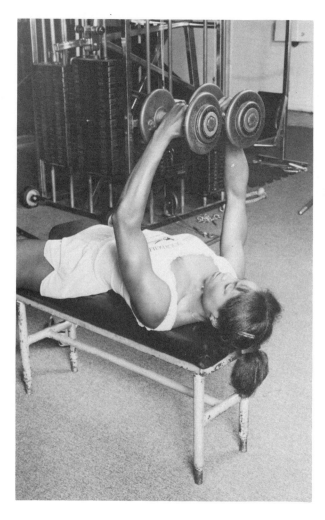

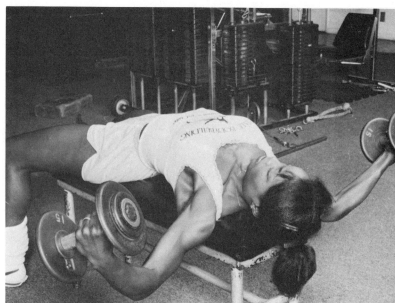

Arms at full outward extension.

Start.

ing sensation in your pectoral muscles. Return the dumbbells along the same semicircular arcs to the starting point of the exercise. Repeat the movement for an appropriate number of repetitions.

Exercise Variations   This movement can also be done on an incline bench to place greater stress on the upper pectoral muscles.

BACK EXERCISES

HYPEREXTENSIONS   Hyperextensions place primary stress on the lower back and hamstring muscles. Second-
Exercise Emphasis   ary stress is placed on the muscles of the buttocks.

Starting Position   Most public gyms have a special bench on which you can do hyperextensions. Stand in the middle of the bench facing the large pad set at about waist height. Lean forward onto this pad, allowing your heels to come to rest beneath the two small pads behind you. Straighten your legs and bend at the waist until your torso is perpendicular to the floor. Interlace your fingers behind your neck and keep your hands in this position throughout
90   the movement.

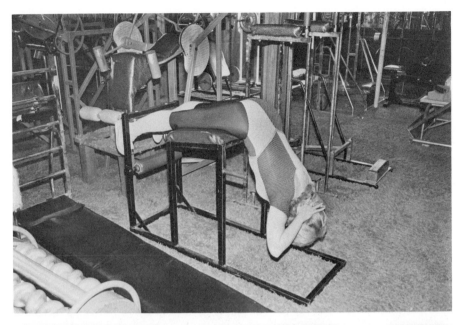

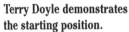

Terry Doyle demonstrates
the starting position.

...and the finish.

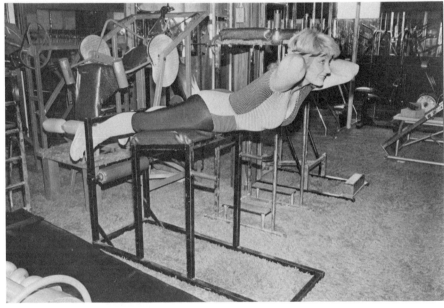

Slowly arch your back to pull your torso upward until it is above an imaginary line drawn parallel to the floor. Hold this top position for a moment, and then allow your torso to return to the starting point of the exercise. Repeat the movement for the required number of repetitions.

Movement Performance

If you don't have a hyperextension bench available, you can still do hyperextensions on a high bench or table with the assistance of a training partner. Simply lie across the table or bench with your torso off of it. With your training partner restraining your legs during the movement, you can comfortably do hyperextensions.

Exercise Variations

Regardless of the variation you perform, you will eventually need to add resistance to the movement. This is most easily done by holding a barbell plate behind your head.

91

UPRIGHT ROWS
Exercise Emphasis

Primary stress in this movement is placed on the deltoids, trapezius muscles, and biceps. Secondary stress is on the forearm muscles. If you have the common posture problem of slightly rounded shoulders, regular use of upright rows in your workout can help to correct it.

Starting Position

Grasp a barbell with your index fingers four to six inches apart. Stand erect with your feet set a comfortable distance apart, and hang your arms down at your sides. In this position, the barbell will rest across your upper thighs, your palms will be toward your body, and your arms will be straight.

Movement Performance

Keeping your elbows above your hands throughout the movement, slowly pull the barbell upward along a plane two or three inches away from your body until the backs of your hands contact your chin. In the top position of the movement, your elbows should be well above the level of your hands, and your shoulders should be rotated slightly to the rear. Slowly lower the bar back to the starting point of the exercise. Repeat the movement for the desired number of reps.

Exercise Variations

You can vary the width of your grip on the barbell. Some bodybuilders feel that a shoulder-width grip places more stress on the deltoids, although most women prefer using a narrow grip on the barbell.

Start. Finish.

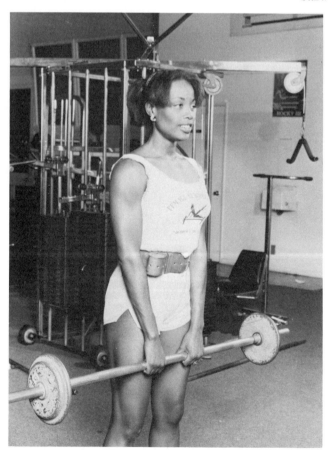
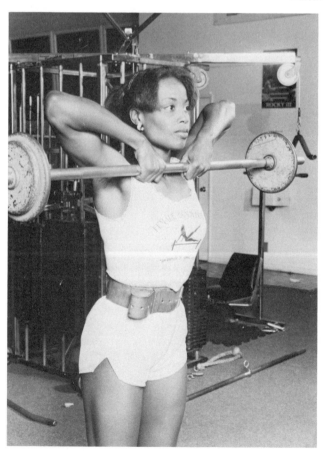

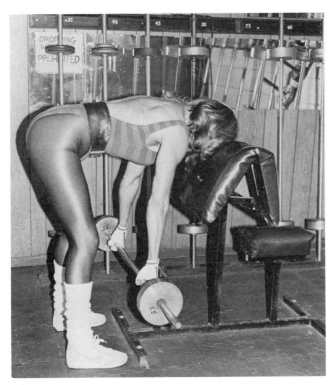 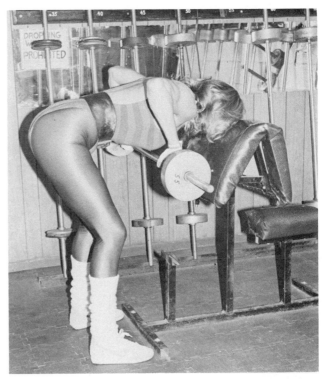

Start.   **Finish.**

Primary stress during barbell bent rows is placed on the latissimus dorsi muscles, the erector spinae muscles of the lower back, and biceps. Secondary stress is placed on the trapezius, brachialis, and forearm muscles.

BARBELL BENT ROWS
Exercise Emphasis

Place your feet at shoulder width a foot or so back from a barbell lying on the floor. Bend over and take a shoulder-width grip on the barbell, with your palms toward your shins. Unlock your knees and keep your legs slightly bent throughout the movement to remove undue stress from the lower back. Arch your back slightly and raise your shoulders until your torso is parallel to the floor. Straighten your arms completely. The barbell plates should now be held just clear of the floor.

Starting Position

Being careful to move your arms slightly to the rear at 45-degree angles from your torso, slowly pull the barbell upward to touch the lower edge of your rib cage. Lower the barbell back to the starting point of the exercise. Repeat the movement for an appropriate number of repetitions.

Movement Performance

As you increase the poundage you use for barbell bent rows, you will inevitably use barbell plates of larger diameter. With large plates, the barbell will still be resting on the floor when your arms are fully extended. Once this happens, you should begin to do your bent rows while standing on either a thick block of wood or the padded surface of a flat exercise bench. With this method, you can use plates of very large diameter without them touching the floor at the bottom of the movement.

Exercise Variations

You can use a wide variety of grip widths when doing barbell bent rows. Many bodybuilders prefer using a grip as much as a foot wider on each side than shoulder width. Many others use a relatively narrow grip with only about six inches of space between the hands. Or, you can use a grip width between these two extremes.

93

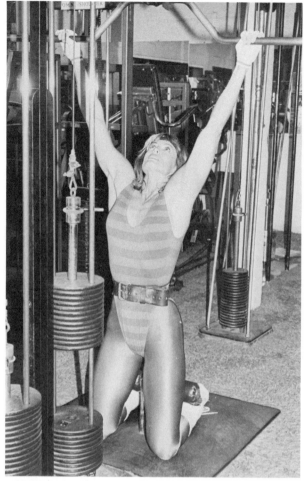

Start.

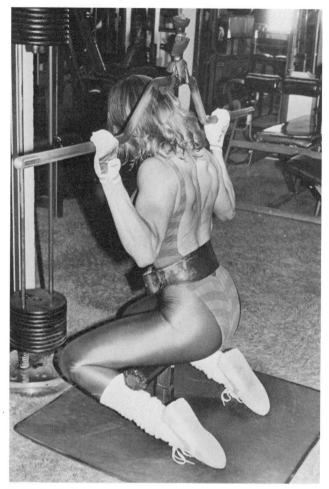

Finish, behind the neck.

LAT MACHINE PULL-DOWNS
Exercise Emphasis

Lat pull-downs primarily stress the latissimus dorsi and biceps muscles. Secondary stress is placed on the brachialis, posterior deltoid, and forearm muscles.

Free-Weight Starting Position

Grasp the lat bar with your palms facing away from your body and your hands set four to six inches wider on each side than the width of your shoulders. Sit on the seat provided directly below the pulley, and wedge your knees under the cross bar above the front edge of the seat. When you are using very heavy weights on your pull-downs, this cross bar will keep your body from rising off the seat. Straighten your arms as fully as possible, and move your shoulders upward toward the pulley to stretch your lats further.

Nautilus Starting Position

Adjust the seat of the machine to a height at which you can sit on it and still fully extend your arms at the top of the movement. Sit on the seat and fasten the belt over your lap to restrain your body in the seat as you do the pull-downs. Grasp the handles of the machine with your palms toward each other, and completely straighten your arms to stretch your lats.

Universal Gyms Starting Position

The starting position on this apparatus is similar in most ways to that on a free-weight lat machine. There is no seat on a Universal machine, however, so you must either sit or kneel directly beneath the pulley of the machine.

Being sure to keep your elbows on a plane slightly behind your torso, slowly pull the bar down to touch the base of your neck behind your head. Allow the bar slowly to return to the starting position. Repeat the movement for an appropriate number of repetitions.

Movement Performance

Rather than pulling the bar down behind your neck, you can pull it down to touch the base of your neck in front of your head. These movements are respectively called pull-downs behind the neck and front pull-downs.

Exercise Variations

There is a huge variety of grips that can be used when doing lat pull-downs. You can face your palms in the opposite direction. And, regardless of the direction you face your palms, you can use any grip width, from one with the hands set a foot or more wider on each side than the width of the shoulders to one in which your hands touch each other in the middle of the bar.

SHOULDER EXERCISES

Military presses place primary stress on the deltoids (particularly the anterior heads of the muscles) and triceps. Secondary stress is on the trapezius and upper pectoral muscle groups.

MILITARY PRESSES
Exercise Emphasis

Stand with your shins up against the bar of a barbell lying on the floor. Bend over and take a shoulder-width grip on the barbell, your palms toward your shins. Flatten your

Starting Position

Start.

Finish.

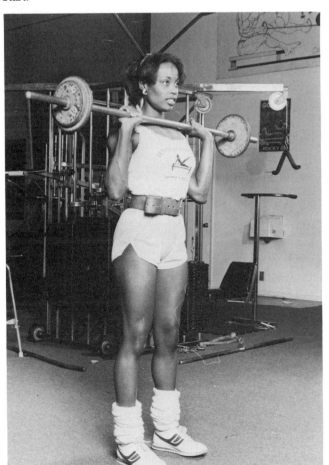
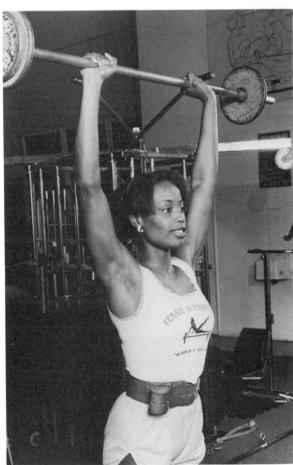

back, dip your hips, and straighten your arms completely. From this position, pull the barbell up to your shoulders by first straightening your legs, then your back. Follow through by pulling with your arms and whipping your elbows under the bar to secure the barbell at your shoulders. This movement, incidentally, is called a power clean. Rotate your elbows downward until they are directly beneath the bar. Stand perfectly erect throughout the movement.

Movement Performance

Making sure not to bend your torso backward, slowly push the barbell directly upward close to your face until it is at straight arm's length directly above your head. Slowly lower the barbell back to your shoulders. Repeat the movement for the required number of repetitions, then return the barbell to the floor.

Exercise Variations

You can use a slightly wider grip when doing military presses. You can also do this movement seated on an exercise bench with your legs locked around the bench to secure your body in position during the movement. Doing seated presses isolates the legs from the exercise, placing more intense stress on the shoulder and triceps muscles.

SIDE LATERAL RAISES
Exercise Emphasis

Often called side laterals, this movement places isolated resistance on the medial head of the deltoids. Minor secondary stress is placed on the front portion of the deltoids and on the trapezius muscles.

Free-Weight
Starting Position

Grasp two light dumbbells and place your feet a comfortable distance apart. Stand erect and bend slightly forward at the waist. Maintain this torso position throughout the movement. With your palms toward each other, press the dumbbells lightly together two or three inches in front of your hips. Bend your arms slightly and keep them bent throughout the movement.

Nautilus Starting
Position

The height of the seat should be at a level that puts your shoulders even with the pivot points of the lever arms of the machine as you sit in the seat. Sit in the seat, cross your legs beneath the seat, and fasten the seat belt over your lap. Place the backs of your wrists against the pads on the movable arms of the machine and lightly grasp the handles near the pads. Move your hands toward each other as far as possible.

Movement Performance

Being careful to keep your elbows at the same level as your hands, slowly raise your hands in semicircular arcs directly out to the sides and upward until your hands are slightly above the level of your shoulders. When using dumbbells, rotate the forward plates downward beneath the level of the back plates at the top of the movement. Slowly lower your hands back to the starting point of the exercise. Repeat the movement for the desired number of reps.

Exercise Variations

This movement can be done with one arm at a time using a dumbbell. Grasp a solid upright with your free hand, and lean slightly toward your working arm when doing one-arm dumbbell side lateral raises.

Start.

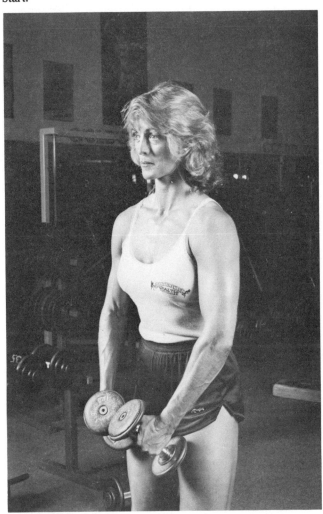

Finish.

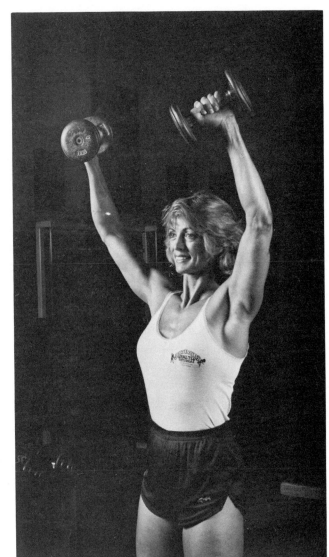

97

ARM EXERCISES

BARBELL CURLS
Exercise Emphasis Barbell curls place primary stress on the biceps and secondary stress on the flexor muscles on the inner sides of your forearms.

Starting Position Take a shoulder-width grip on a barbell, with your palms facing away from your body as you stand erect with your arms down at your sides and the barbell resting across your thighs. Pin your upper arms against the sides of your torso, and keep them in this position throughout the movement.

Movement Performance Slowly bend your arms and move the barbell in a semicircular arc from the tops of your thighs to your shoulders. Be careful not to allow your torso to sway back and forth. Lower the weight back to the starting point, and repeat the movement for an appropriate number of repetitions.

Exercise Variations If you have trouble keeping your torso motionless, you can do barbell curls with your back resting against a wall. You can also experiment with wider and narrower grips on the bar.

Patsy Chapman demonstrates the starting position.

...and the finish.

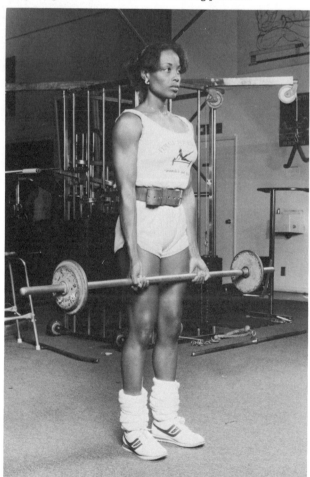
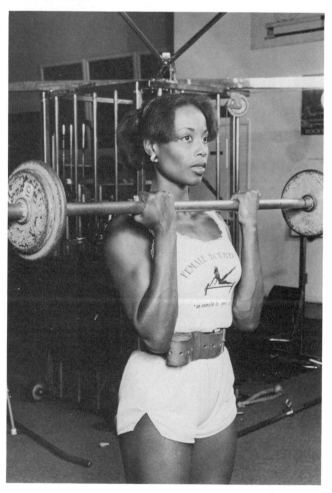

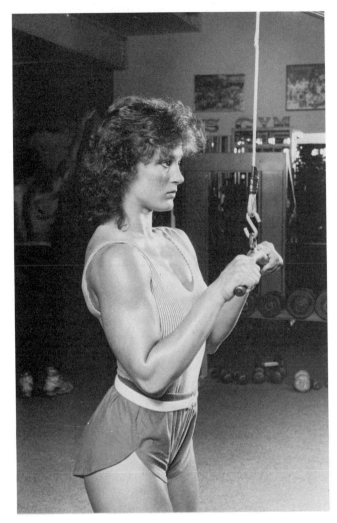

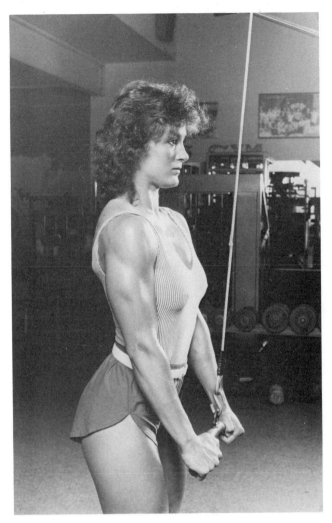

Start.   Finish.

Push-downs place primary stress on the triceps muscles and secondary stress on the flexor muscles of the forearms.

Stand facing a lat machine bar, your toes about a foot back from a point directly beneath the bar. Grasp the bar with your palms facing away from your body and your hands about six inches apart. Pull the bar down far enough so you can pin your upper arms against the sides of your torso throughout the movement. Fully bend your arms.

Starting Position

Slowly straighten your arms fully. Hold this position for a moment, then slowly allow the weight to return your arms to the starting point of the exercise. Repeat the movement for the required number of repetitions.

Movement Performance

There are several types of handles that you can use when performing push-downs. With a long, straight bar, you can use wider grips. Most contemporary bodybuilders, however, prefer to use a short bar handle that is bent in the middle so each grip angles downward at the end. Some women prefer to use a handle consisting of two stands of rope hanging from the cable. This rope handle allows you to do push-downs with your palms toward each other. (This is called a "parallel grip.")

Exercise Variations

99

Start of regular wrist curls.

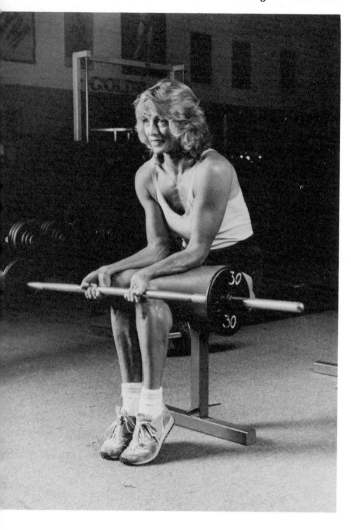

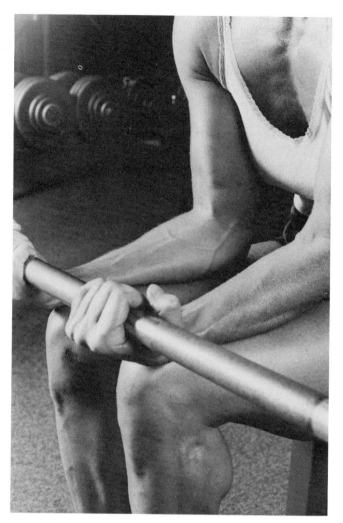

Finish.

BARBELL WRIST CURLS/REVERSE WRIST CURLS
Exercise Emphasis

When done with palms up, wrist curls stress the flexor muscles on the insides of the forearms. Done with palms down, reverse wrist curls stress the extensor muscles on the outsides of the forearms.

Starting Position

Sit at the end of a flat exercise bench and position your feet on the floor, set apart at shoulder width. Take a shoulder-width grip on the barbell so that your palms are facing upward in the starting position of the movement. Run your forearms down your thighs so your wrists and fists hang off the edges of your knees. Sag your fists as far toward the floor as possible.

Start of reverse wrist curls.

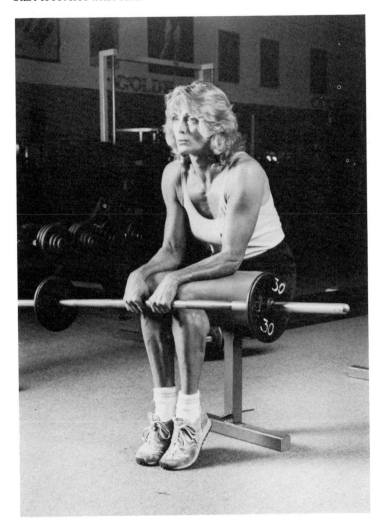

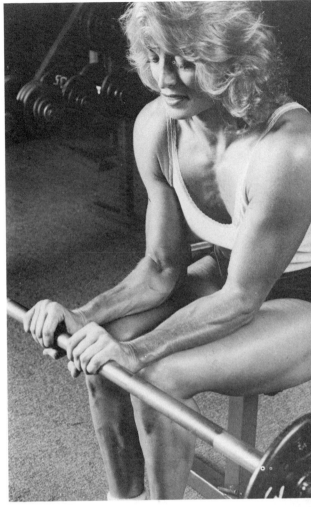

Finish.

Movement Performance

Slowly curl the barbell upward in a small semicircular arc as high as possible by flexing your wrists. Lower the barbell back to the starting point of the exercise, and repeat the movement for the desired number of repetitions.

Exercise Variations

Of course, you can do reverse wrist curls with your palms down. You will find that you can use only about half as much weight with your palms down as with your palms up. Regardless of whether you do the movement with your palms up or down, you can experiment with both narrow and wide grip widths.

101

CALF EXERCISES

STANDING BARBELL CALF RAISE
Exercise Emphasis

This is a simple movement that stresses the gastrocnemius muscles of the calves.

Starting Position

Place a moderately weighted barbell behind your neck and across your shoulders as though preparing to do a set of squats. Place your toes and the balls of your feet on a 4 × 4-inch block of wood, which will allow you to stretch your calves better during the movement, since your heels can be lowered considerably below the level of your toes when using such a block. Your feet should be set about shoulder-width apart, and your toes should be directly forward. Lower your heels as far as possible below the level of your toes.

Movement Performance

Slowly rise up on your toes as high as you can. Lower your heels slowly back to the starting point of the exercise. Repeat the movement for the required number of repetitions. You will find it difficult to balance your body in position during this exercise, which is the reason why experienced bodybuilders use a standing calf machine to perform a similar movement. I have included this movement for women who train at home and don't have access to a standing calf machine.

Exercise Variations

On all calf exercises, you should use three different toe positions to stress your calf muscles from several angles. You should do some of your sets with your toes pointed straight

Start.

Finish (close-up).

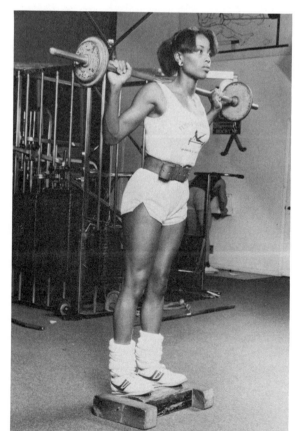

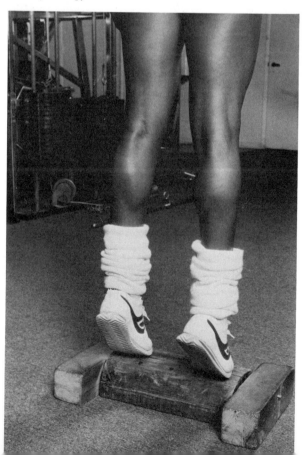

ahead, some with your feet angled outward at 45 degrees on each side, and some with your feet pointed inward at 45-degree angles. You can also vary the width of your toe placement on the wooden block on most of your calf exercises.

Standing toe raises on a calf machine provide very direct stress to the gastrocnemius muscles of the calves, but without balance problems.

STANDING CALF MACHINE TOE RAISES
Exercise Emphasis

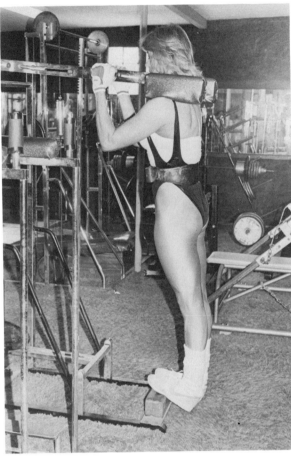 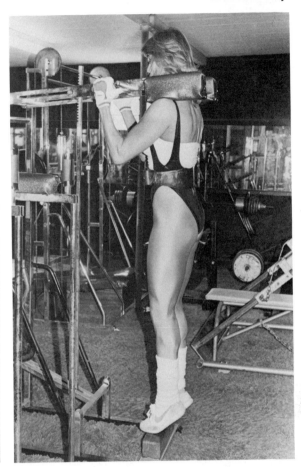

Start.   Finish.

Bend your legs enough so you can rest the yokes of the machine over your shoulders. Place your toes and the balls of your feet on the calf block, with your feet set at shoulder width and your toes pointed directly ahead. Straighten your legs and body completely, and keep them straight throughout the movement. Sag your heels as far below the level of your toes as possible to fully stretch your calf muscles.

Starting Position

Slowly rise up as high as possible on your toes. Lower your heels slowly back down to the starting point of the exercise. Repeat the movement for an appropriate number of repetitions.

Movement Performance

Be sure to use all three recommended toe positions on this exercise, and occasionally change the width of your foot placement on the block.

Exercise Variations

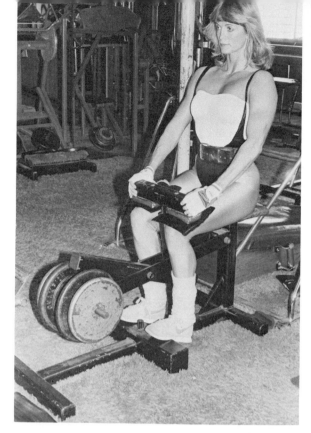

Start.

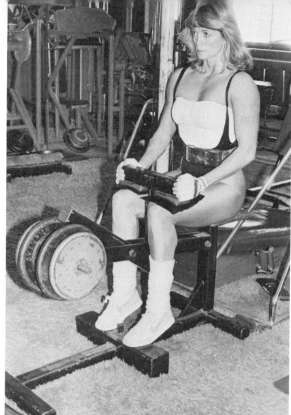

Finish.

Exercise Emphasis

This movement strongly stresses the wide, thin soleus muscle that lies beneath the gastrocnemius. The soleus gives width to the calf when it is viewed from the front or back. The soleus can only be fully contracted when the leg is bent at an approximate 90-degree angle, so seated toe raises are the only movement that will fully develop the muscle.

Starting Position

This exercise is normally done on a special seated calf machine. Sit on the machine's seat and place your toes and the balls of your feet on the toe plate, with your toes pointed directly forward. By removing a pin in the column of steel that attaches the weight to pads that rest over your knees, you can adjust these pads to a height that allows you to slip your knees under them while your feet are on the toe plate. Rise up on your toes two or three inches, and push the movable stop bar of the machine forward to release the weight. Sag your heels as far below the level of your toes as possible.

Movement Performance

Slowly extend your toes as completely as possible, pushing your knees against the pads and raising them as high as possible. Slowly allow your heels to sink back to the starting point of the exercise. Repeat the movement for the required number of repetitions. Lock the stop bar at the end of your set.

Exercise Variations

If you don't have access to a seated calf machine, you can still do this exercise with a barbell, towel, wooden calf block, and flat exercise bench. Place the calf block about eighteen inches from the end of the bench. Place the barbell on the floor between the block and bench, load it up with a moderately heavy weight, and wrap the towel around the middle of the bar to pad it enough so it won't cut into your knees. Pull the barbell up and rest the bar on your knees. Sit down on the bench with the barbell still resting on your

104

knees, then position your toes and the balls of your feet on the calf block. You can do a very effective seated calf raise once you are in this position.

Regardless of the variation of seated calf raises that you perform, use all three recommended toe positions, and occasionally vary the width of your foot placement on the toe plate or calf block.

MIDSECTION EXERCISES

Sit-ups stress the frontal abdominal wall, particularly the upper half of the rectus abdominis muscle group.

SIT-UPS
Exercise Emphasis

Lie on your back on the floor or on an adjustable abdominal board with your feet toward either a heavy piece of furniture or the end of the abdominal board with roller pads. Slip your feet under the piece of furniture if you are lying on the floor or under the roller pads if you are lying on an abdominal board. In both cases, bend your legs at approximately a 30-degree angle to remove potentially harmful stress from your lower back. Place your hands behind your neck or head, and interlace your fingers to keep them in this position throughout the movement.

Starting Position

Slowly curl your torso from the floor, lifting first your head and shoulders, then the middle of your back, and finally the small of your back until your torso is perpendicular to

Movement Performance

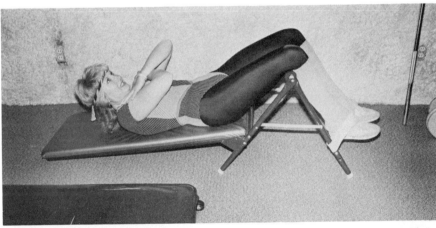

Terry Doyle demonstrates the starting position.

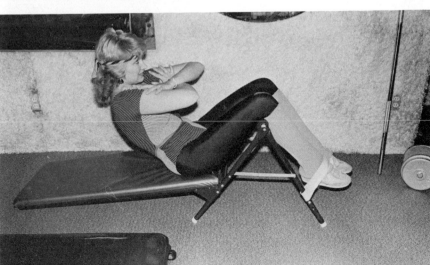

...and the finish.

the floor. Reverse the procedure to lower your torso back to the starting point of the exercise. Repeat the movement for the desired number of repetitions.

Exercise Variations   If you are doing your sit-ups on an abdominal board, you can make the exercise more intense by raising the foot end of the board. On all variations of sit-ups, you can involve the intercostal muscles by twisting alternately to each side on successive reps.

LEG RAISES
Exercise Emphasis   Leg raises stress the frontal abdominal wall, particularly the lower half of the rectus abdominis muscle group.

Starting Position   Lie on your back on either the floor or an abdominal board, but with your feet in the opposite direction from that used when doing sit-ups. Grasp either the heavy piece of furniture or the roller pads behind your head throughout the movement. Bend your legs slightly to remove stress from your lower back, and keep them bent throughout the movement.

Movement Performance   Slowly raise your feet in a semicircular arch from the floor or abdominal board to a position directly above your pelvis. Lower your feet back to the starting point of the exercise, and repeat the movement for an appropriate number of repetitions.

Start.

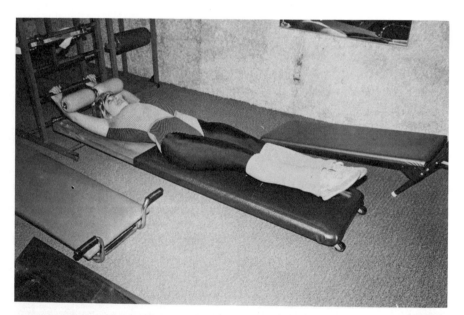

Finish.

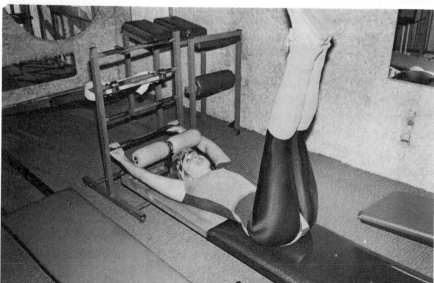

You can make the exercise more intense by raising the head end of the abdominal board. For an interesting effect on your abdominal muscles, try doing the movement without allowing your feet to touch the floor or abdominal board at the end of each repetition. This technique keeps continuous tension on the abdominals, which stresses them quite intensely.

Exercise Variations

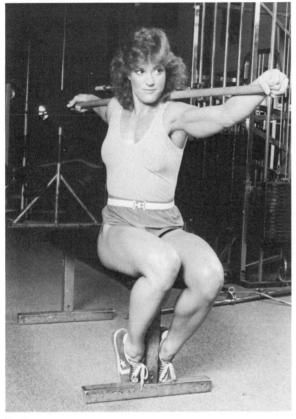
Start.

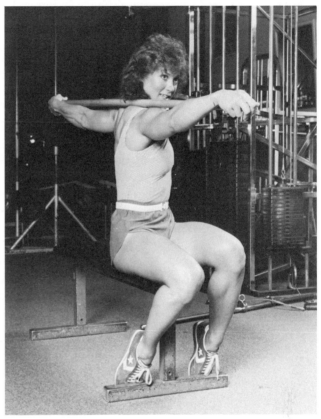
Finish.

This movement stresses and firms the external oblique muscles at the sides of the waist. It also helps to realign the lumbar vertebrae of the lower back.

SEATED TWISTING
Exercise Emphasis

Sit near the end of a flat exercise bench in a position where you can lock your feet in the supports of the bench to restrain your legs and hips during the movement. Place a broomstick across your shoulders behind your neck, and wrap your arms around it.

Starting Position

Forcefully twist your shoulders and torso as far as you can to the left, then immediately twist back as far as possible to the right. Twist quickly from side to side for the required number of repetitions, counting one full cycle from left to right and back to the left again as a single rep.

Movement Performance

This movement is frequently done while standing erect, but very few women perform it correctly in this position. To be effective, standing twists must be done with the pelvis held stationary. Unfortunately, most women who do the standing movement twist their pelvis from side to side along with their torsos and shoulders.

Exercise Variations

107

LEVEL ONE WORKOUTS

Each of the three workouts presented in this section can be followed for four to six weeks before progressing to the next level of intensity. Your individual temperament will dictate how long you remain on a particular workout. If you tend to become easily bored by routine tasks, change training programs each four weeks. (A handful of successful bodybuilders change their routines each workout day.) More stoic women can successfully follow a suggested workout for six or more weeks, particularly in the advanced stages of training.

As you begin using the initial training program, be careful to follow the gradual muscle break-in procedure outlined in Chapter 3. Overly enthusiastic beginning bodybuilders often attempt to train too hard and with excessively heavy weights, which will lead to severe muscle soreness. Remember that weight training is a much more intense form of muscular exercise than anything you've previously experienced. Therefore, a gradual break-in to heavy bodybuilding workouts is mandatory.

After many years of research and experimentation on my own body, I have concluded that an advanced bodybuilder—one who has learned to train very intensely within every set of each exercise she performs—needs to do fewer total sets each workout than less experienced trainees. Level One bodybuilders must learn to perform every exercise *correctly, gradually* increase the total number of sets they do for each muscle group, and *slowly* add to the poundage they use in each movement.

This trend will continue through Level Two, until your muscles are strong enough and your cardio-respiratory efficiency is good enough for you to begin using a variety of training intensification techniques. Then you will systematically decrease the total number of sets you perform for each muscle group in a workout.

It is axiomatic in bodybuilding training that *the greater the intensity of each set for a particular muscle group, the less total sets you can perform for that muscle.* This principle is the same in running—the faster you run, the less distance you can cover at that pace. A good woman sprinter will run 100 meters in a bit more than eleven seconds, while a world-class 1500-meter runner will require an additional five seconds to run each 100 meters of her race.

If you graph the total number of sets you do for your entire body through beginning, intermediate, and advanced stages of bodybuilding training, the peak of the curve will be during Level Two (see Figure 1). The curve on a graph of training intensity, however, will still be rising in Level Three (see Figure 2). Note that these two graphs represent an "average" woman. One or both of your own graphs will probably look somewhat different. In Figure 2, the "Units of Intensity" are totally arbitrary.

108

FIGURE 1: TOTAL TRAINING VOLUME

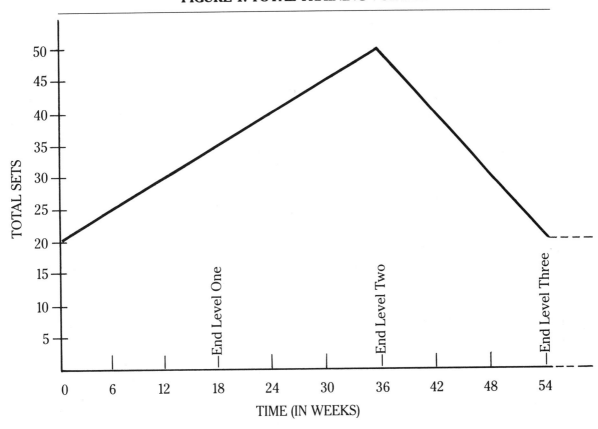

FIGURE 2: TRAINING INTENSITY

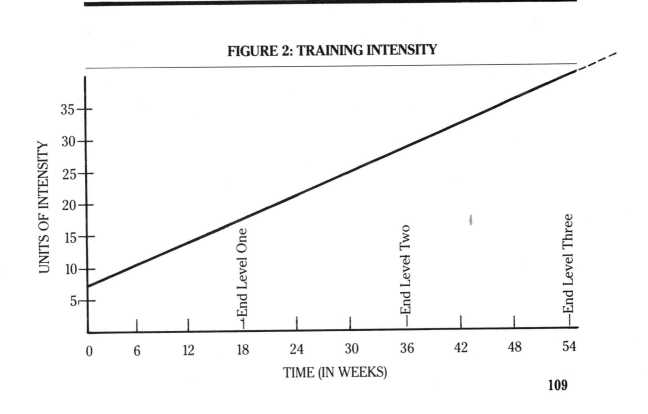

FIRST LEVEL ONE WORKOUT

Use this workout for four to six weeks. Be careful to use correct exercise form and follow the recommended break-in procedure. Only after your muscles are fully accustomed to handling the heavier load of weight training should you begin to concentrate on adding resistance to each exercise.

MONDAY/WEDNESDAY/FRIDAY

Exercise	Sets	Reps	% Body Weight*
1. Sit-ups	1	15–30	0%
2. Seating twisting	1	30–50	0%
3. Leg extensions	3	10–15	25%
4. Leg curls	2	10–15	15%
5. Bench press	3	8–12	25%
6. Lat machine pull-downs	3	8–12	30%
7. Military presses	2	8–12	25%
8. Barbell curls	2	8–12	25%
9. Barbell wrist curls	2	10–15	20%
10. Standing calf machine toe raises	3	15–20	35%

*This refers to the recommended weight to use with exercises employing weights or weight machine resistance.

You will notice that I have not included exercises in this workout for the neck and triceps muscles. I know of no woman bodybuilder who performs direct neck exercises, since the neck muscles grow sufficiently strong and well toned merely from doing upper back and shoulder movements. At the beginning level, your triceps muscles will be sufficiently stimulated by bench presses and military presses.

SECOND LEVEL ONE WORKOUT

There will be several new exercises to master in this workout. Since you won't be required to follow a break-in procedure at this point, you can concentrate more on adding resistance to each of your exercises. Be careful not to sacrifice strict exercise form merely to use five additional pounds in a movement, however. Advanced bodybuilders are able to "cheat" on an exercise to subject the working muscles to even greater intensity. Beginners invariably cheat to remove resistance from a muscle.

I won't suggest starting weights for exercises from this point onward. After four to six weeks of regular workouts, you will have a much better feel for your own strength levels than I could ever have.

MONDAY/WEDNESDAY/FRIDAY

Exercise	Sets	Reps
1. Leg raises	2–3	20–30
2. Side bends	2–3	30–50
3. Lunges	2	10–15
4. Leg extensions	2	10–15
5. Leg curls	3	10–15
6. Incline presses	3	8–12
7. Flat-bench flyes	2	8–12
8. Barbell bent rows	3	8–12
9. Upright rows	2	8–12

MONDAY/WEDNESDAY/FRIDAY (con't.)

Exercise	Sets	Reps
10. Side laterals	3	8–12
11. Barbell curls	2	8–12
12. Pulley push-downs	2	8–12
13. Barbell wrist curls	2	10–15
14. Barbell reverse wrist curls	2	10–15
15A. Seated calf machine toe raises	4	10–15
15B. Standing calf machine toe raises	4	15–20

NOTE: Alternate exercises 15A and 15B each successive workout. Or, you can do both movements every training session, but perform only two sets of each.

Again, there will be several new movements to master in this workout, most notably the squats. And, as with the previous routine, you will be required to do a few additional total sets. Longer workouts are more fatiguing, which spawns the temptation to take longer rest intervals between sets. A well-conditioned bodybuilder could easily complete the following workout in forty-five to fifty minutes. If you take more than sixty minutes to finish the workout, you are training too slowly and allowing your body to cool down. Never rest longer than sixty seconds between sets.

THIRD LEVEL ONE WORKOUT

MONDAY/WEDNESDAY/FRIDAY

Exercise	Sets	Reps
1. Sit-ups	2	20–30
2. Leg raises	2	20–30
3. Seated twisting	2	50
4. Squats	3	10–15
5. Leg extensions	2	10–15
6. Leg curls	3	10–15
7. Incline presses	3	8–12
8. Flat-bench flyes	3	8–12
9. Hyperextensions	2	10–15
10. Barbell bent rows	3	8–12
11. Upright rows	2	8–12
12. Military presses	3	8–12
13. Side laterals	2	8–12
14. Barbell curls	3	8–12
15. Pulley push-downs	3	8–12
16. Barbell wrist curls	2	10–15
17. Barbell reverse wrist curls	2	10–15
18A. Standing calf machine toe raises	5	15–20
18B. Seated calf machine toe raises	5	10–15

NOTE: Alternate exercises 18A and 18B each successive workout. Alternatively, do both 18A and 18B (two or three sets of each) in the same training session.

LEVEL TWO WORKOUTS | 7

At this point you should be seeing positive changes in your physical appearance, muscle tone, and strength from week to week. The speed at which you make such improvements, however, will be highly individual.

Your genetic potential for developing strength and building firm muscle tissue—plus the intensity and regularity with which you train—are responsible for the speed at which you make bodybuilding gains. And, if you ultimately decide to become a competitive bodybuilder, your genetic potential will set the limits to which you can develop your muscles.

Some women are genetically gifted bodybuilders, others are not. Most women fall along a continuum between these two extremes. Less than 5 percent of all women can be considered either genetically gifted or cursed as bodybuilders, so chances are good that you fall into the large group of women who have only "average" potential for success in the sport.

While genetic potential does play a role in bodybuilding, it is not the limiting factor that many competitors make it out to be. Instead, the desire and ability to train consistently at 100 percent effort and maintain a good diet are the keys to success.

I have frequently seen women with very poor genetic potential for bodybuilding succeed handsomely through great dedication to the sport. It can be done, so don't make the excuse of having poor potential. Instead of crying about it, overcome it!

THIGH AND HIP EXERCISES

LEG PRESSES
Exercise Emphasis

Like squats, leg presses stress all of the thigh, buttock, and hip muscles, particularly the quadriceps on the fronts of the thighs. Unlike squats, no strain is placed on the lower back, so you can safely do leg presses even when your lower back is sore.

113

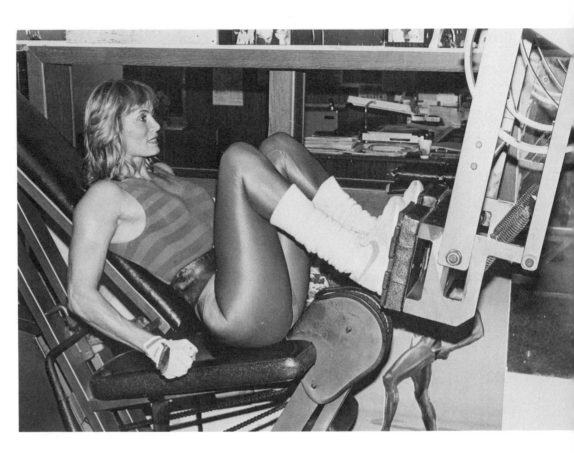

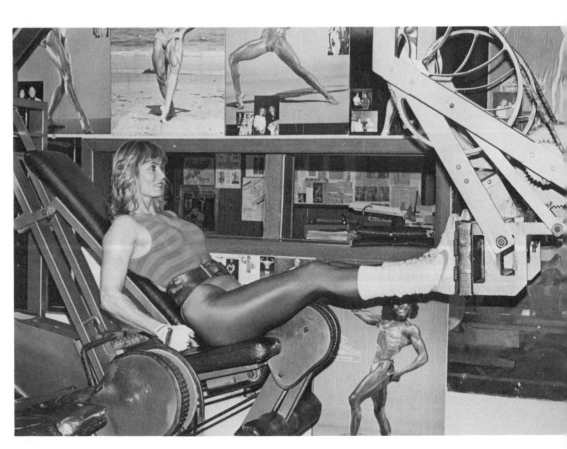

114

Lie on your back beneath the machine's sliding platform, and place your hips at the upper end of the angled pad directly beneath the platform. Bend your legs and place your feet at shoulder width on the sliding platform. Straighten your legs. Rotate the machine's stop bars to release the sliding platform during the movement.

Free-Weight Starting Position (Vertical Machine)

Sit with your hips in the angle formed by the back and seat pads of the machine, and lie back against the angled backrest. Bend your legs and place your feet at shoulder width on the sliding platform. Straighten your legs. Rotate the machine's stop bars to release the sliding platform during the movement.

Free-Weight Starting Position (45-Degree Machine)

Sit on the seat of the Nautilus double leg machine, and adjust the backrest forward so your legs are fully bent when you place your feet on the movement platforms. You can adjust the backrest by pulling up on a handle near your hips on the right side of the machine, then pulling the backrest forward as much as needed. Once you have the backrest in the desired position, simply lower the handle to lock it into position. Place your feet against the movement platforms, and grasp the handles at the sides of your hips to hold your body in position throughout the movement. Straighten your legs.

Nautilus Starting Position

Adjust the seat of the machine so your legs are fully bent when you place your feet on the movement pedals. You can adjust the seat by pulling up on the knob at the front edge, sliding the seat forward or backward to the appropriate position, and releasing the knob to lock the seat in place. Sit in the seat, bend your legs, and place your feet on the pedals. Grasp the handles at the sides of your hips and straighten your legs. Be sure to keep your torso erect throughout the movement, since slumping your shoulders forward can place your upper back in a position where it is open to injury.

Universal Gyms Starting Position

Slowly bend your legs as fully as possible, then straighten them to within a few degrees of a fully straight position. Repeat the movement for desired number of repetitions.

Movement Performance

On the two free-weight leg press machines, you can vary the width of your foot placement on the platforms. On the Nautilus and Universal machines, you can vary your foot angle, placing your feet straight ahead, angling your toes outward, or angling your toes inward. Each variation of foot placement affects your thigh muscles a bit differently.

Exercise Variations

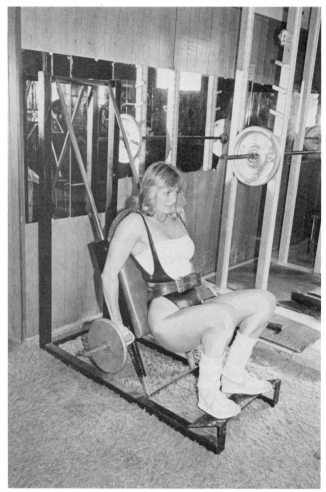

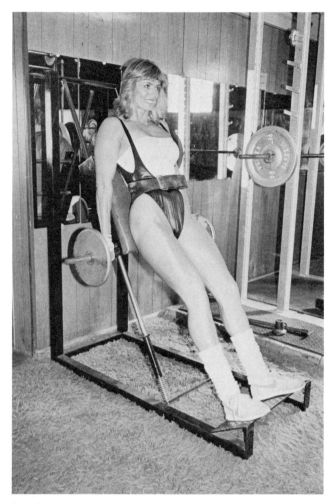

In the squat position. **Legs fully extended.**

HACK MACHINE Hacks stress the frontal thigh muscles—particularly those just above the knees—in relative
SQUATS isolation from the rest of the body. Minor secondary stress is placed on the hamstrings
Exercise Emphasis and buttocks.

Platform-type Starting Bend your legs and place your back flat against the movable platform of the machine.
Position Grasp the handles attached to the bottom edge of the platform, and place your feet at
about shoulder width on the angled foot rest. Straighten your legs and throw your head
slightly back.

Yoke-type Starting A type of hack machine with only yokes that fit over the shoulders is becoming more
Position and more popular. Rest your shoulders beneath the yokes, and place your feet about
shoulder width apart on the angled foot rest. Straighten your legs and rotate the machine's
stop bars to release the sliding part of the machine for movement.

Movement Performance Slowly bend your legs as fully as possible under resistance, then straighten them completely. Repeat the movement for the required number of repetitions.

Exercise Variations You can use the same variations of stance width and toe angles as for leg presses.

The movement done on a Nautilus hip and back machine strongly stresses the buttocks and erector spinae muscles.

Lie on your back with your knees resting over the movement roller pads and your hips as near the edge of the bench toward the pivot points of the machine as possible. Most Nautilus hip and back machines have a small portable pad on which you should rest your head and neck during the movement. Fasten the lap belt across your hips, and grasp the handles at the sides of your hips to steady your body in position throughout the movement. Push down with your knees slowly to straighten your body and arch your back.

Starting Position

Keeping your right leg in line with your torso, slowly allow your left knee to move in a semicircular arc to a position as close to your chest as is comfortably possible. Use your buttock and lower back strength to return your knee to the starting position. Repeat the movement with your right leg, and alternate legs until you have done the required number of repetitions with each leg.

Movement Performance

By holding the position with your entire body in one straight line for a few seconds between each repetition, you can achieve a valuable peak contraction effect in the working muscles. You can also work one leg at a time for an appropriate number of reps while keeping the other leg in line with your torso.

Exercise Variations

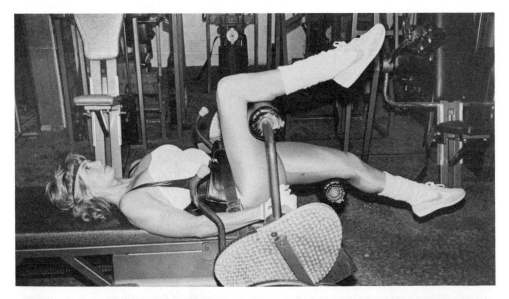

Right leg up, left leg extended.

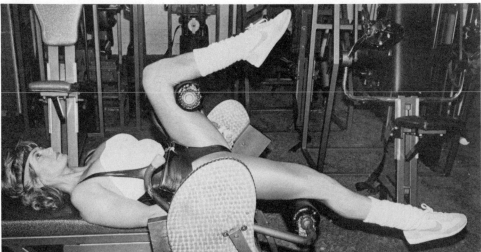

Left leg up, right leg extended.

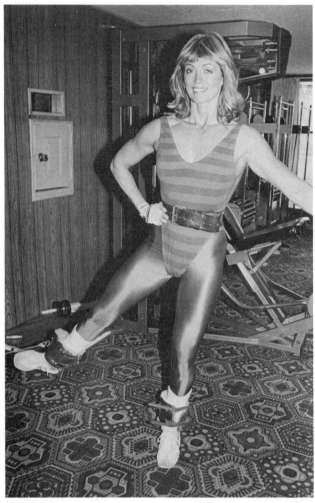 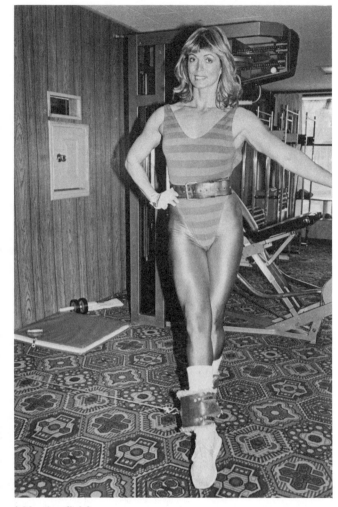

Adduction start.   Adduction finish.

CABLE LEG ADDUC-
TION/ABDUCTION
Exercise Emphasis

Cable leg adductions stress the inner thigh muscles, while adbuctions stress the muscles on the sides of your thighs and hips.

Adduction Starting
Position

Use an ankle cuff to attach the end of a cable running through a floor pulley to your right ankle. Stand erect with your right side far enough away from the pulley to keep resistance on your working leg throughout the movement. Grasp a sturdy upright to retain balance throughout the movement, and allow your right foot to travel as far out to the side as possible. Hold your right leg straight throughout the movement.

Adduction Movement
Performance

118

Using the muscles of your inner thighs, slowly pull your working leg inward until it touches the leg on which you are supporting your weight. Allow the cable force to pull your working foot back to the starting point and repeat the movement. Do the same number of sets and reps for each leg.

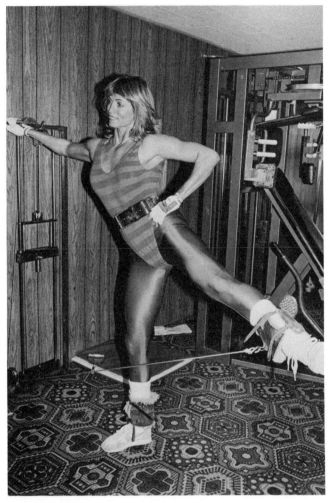

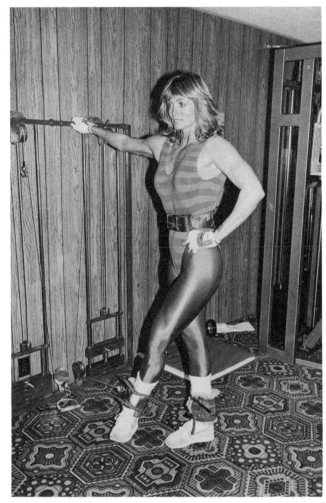

Abduction start.   Abduction finish.

Fasten the cable to your right foot as for an adduction movement, but with your left *Adbuction Starting*
side toward the pulley and the cable running across the plane of your body. Grasp *Position*
a sturdy upright for balance during the movement. Allow the weight of the apparatus
to pull your right leg well across the midline of your body. Keep your working leg
straight during the movement.

Using the muscles of your upper thighs and hips, slowly pull your working leg across *Abduction Movement*
your body and out to the side as far as possible, then allow the weight to pull the foot *Performance*
back to the starting point of the movement. Repeat the movement for the desired number
of sets and repetitions. Be sure to do the same number of sets and repetitions for each leg.

Many women like to do this exercise either directly facing the pulley and pulling the work- *Exercise Variations*
ing leg backward or facing the pulley and moving the working leg forward. The first of
these variations stresses the quadriceps muscles, the second primarily the muscles of the
buttocks and hips.   **119**

CHEST EXERCISES

MACHINE FLYES
Exercise Emphasis
Performed on a Nautilus machine, this movement stresses the lower and inner sections of the pectoral muscles. Done on a free-weight pec deck, it stresses the entire pectoral muscle, particularly its inner edges.

Nautilus Starting Position
Adjust the seat of the machine to a level so your upper arms are parallel to the floor throughout the movement. Sit in the seat and fasten the lap belt over your hips. Place your elbows against the movable pads of the machine, and grasp the handles attached to the pads. Keep your head back against the machine's backrest throughout the movement.

Pec Deck Starting Position
Adjust the seat of the machine to a height that keeps your upper arms parallel to the floor during the movement. Sit on the seat and rest your elbows and forearms against the pads, with your forearms perpendicular to the floor. Keep your head back against the machine's vertical backrest during the movement, and allow your elbows to travel as far to the rear as possible.

Movement Performance
Using your pectoral strength, push against the pads with your elbows to move them inward to touch each other directly in front of your chest. Hold this fully contracted position for two or three seconds to achieve a peak contraction effect in your pecs. Then slowly allow the pads to return to the starting position. Repeat for an appropriate number of repetitions.

Nautilus starting position.

Finish, with training partner assisting on a forced rep.

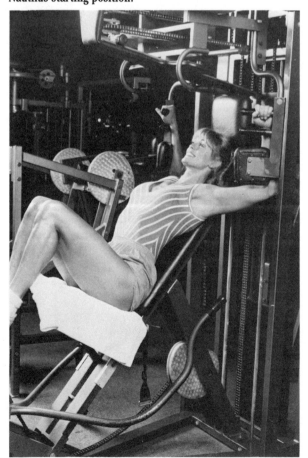
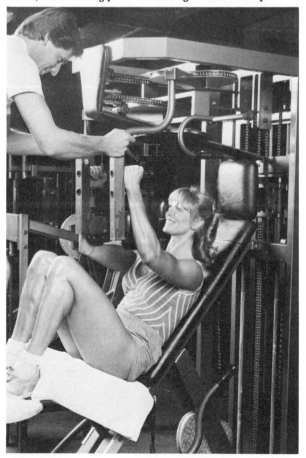

You can use either type of equipment to do the movement with one arm at a time. Doing any exercise with one arm or leg at a time allows you to place greater than normal concentration on the working muscles.

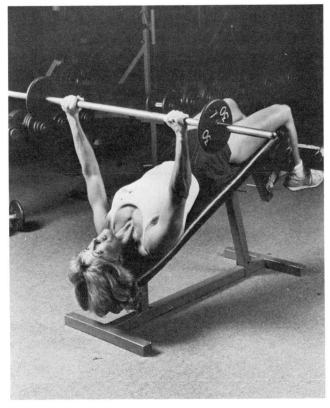

Start, using a wide grip.

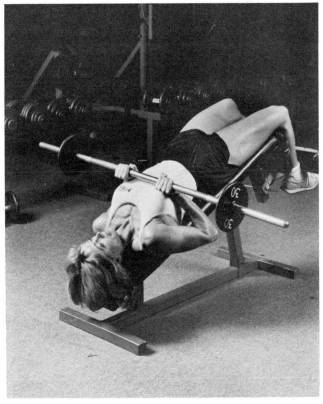

Finish, showing a narrow grip.

All chest movements done on a decline bench place major stress on the lower third of the pectoral muscle complex. Decline presses also strongly stress the front portion of the deltoids and the triceps. Secondary emphasis is placed on the latissimus dorsi muscles.

DECLINE BARBELL PRESS
Exercise Emphasis

Lie back on a decline bench, with your head at the lower end, and brace your feet under the bench's toe bar to keep your body from sliding down the bench during the movement. Take a grip with your hands set four or five inches wider than your shoulders on each side, your palms toward your feet. Straighten your arms and lift the barbell off the rack. At the starting point, the barbell will be directly above your shoulder joints. From the sides, your arms will appear to be perpendicular to the floor.

Starting Position

Being sure to hold your elbows back as much as you can, slowly bend your arms and lower the barbell down until it touches the lower part of your rib cage. Press the barbell back to the starting point, and repeat the movement for the desired number of reps.

Movement Performance

As with all variations of the barbell bench press, you can vary the width of your grip on the bar. You can also do decline presses on decline benches set at a variety of angles or on a flat exercise bench with a 4 × 4-inch block of wood placed under the foot end of the bench.

Exercise Variations

121

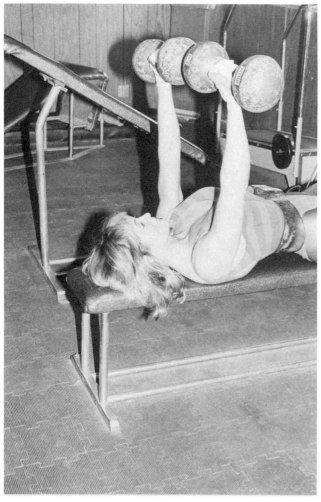

Arms at full extension.

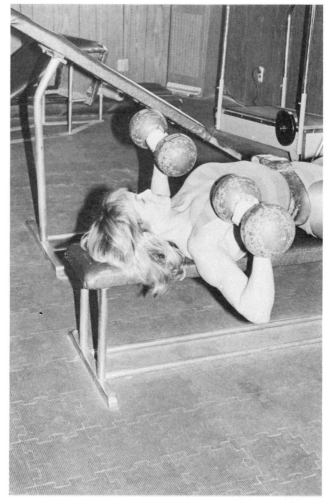

Arms in position to press weights back up.

DUMBBELL BENCH PRESSES *Exercise Emphasis*	All forms of dumbbell bench presses strongly stress the pectorals, deltoids, and triceps. Incline dumbbell presses stress the upper pectorals more strongly than flat-bench dumbbell presses, while decline dumbbell presses shift emphasis more to the lower pectorals.
Starting Position	Grasp two moderately weighted dumbbells, and lie back on a flat, incline, or decline bench. Push the dumbbells to straight arm's length directly above your shoulder joints. Your palms should be facing forward, and the dumbbells should be touching each other directly above your chest.
Movement Performance	Keeping your elbows back, slowly bend your arms and lower the dumbbells down to a point slightly below the level of your shoulders. Press the dumbbells back to the starting point, and repeat the movement for an appropriate number of repetitions.
Exercise Variations	You can also do this movement with your palms facing each other rather than directly forward. You can use a variety of incline and decline bench angles as well.

Dips strongly stress the lower pectorals, the front portion of the deltoids, and the triceps.

Grasp a pair of parallel bars with your palms facing each other, and jump to a supported position on straight arms above the bars. Bend your legs at 90-degree angles and cross your ankles. Bend slightly at the waist so your torso is angled slightly forward at your shoulders.

Starting Position

Allowing your elbows to move slightly to the rear, slowly bend your arms and lower your body as far below the level of the bars as possible. Push yourself back to the starting point, and repeat the movement for the desired number of repetitions.

Movement Performance

If you do this movement with your torso held erect rather than inclined forward, you put more stress on your frontal deltoid and triceps muscles. In many gyms you will find bars that are angled inward at the ends. These bars allow you to take different grip widths when doing parallel bar dips. Once you can comfortably do at least ten repetitions of dips, you can hang a dumbbell around your waist with a specially designed dip belt.

Exercise Variations

Start.

Finish.

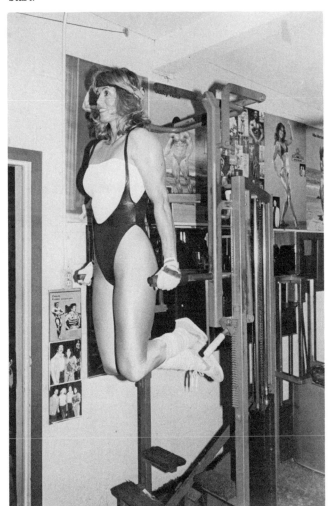
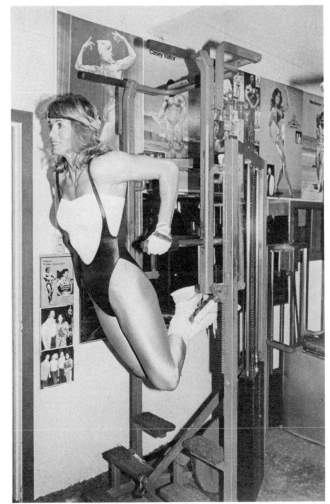

BACK EXERCISES

BARBELL SHRUGS
Exercise Emphasis — Shrugs place direct stress on the trapezius muscles of your upper back. Minor secondary stress is placed on the flexor muscles of your forearms.

Starting Position — Grasp a heavy barbell with a shoulder-width grip, your palms toward your legs. Stand erect with your arms straight and the barbell resting across your upper thighs. Sag your shoulders downward and forward as far as comfortably possible.

Movement Performance — Slowly shrug your shoulders upward and backward as high as you can, then lower the weight back to the starting point. Repeat the movement for the required number of repetitions.

Exercise Variations — For a slightly different effect on your trapezius muscles, you can take a wider grip. Many advanced bodybuilders prefer to load up the barbell and place it on a flat exercise bench, from which it can be lifted up to the starting point of the movement.

Start.

Finish.

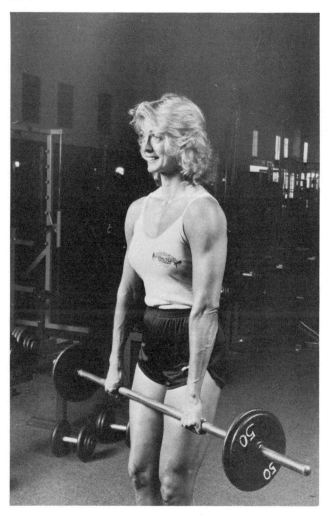

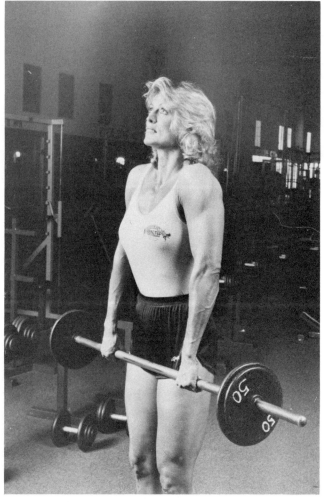

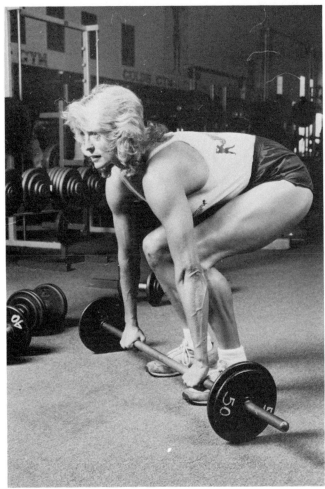

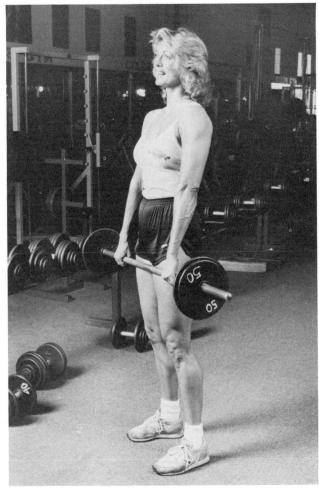

Start.   Finish.

Deadlifts place heavy stress on the lower back, hip, buttock, and quadriceps muscles. Secondary stress is placed on the upper back, abdominal, and forearm muscles.

DEADLIFTS
Exercise Emphasis

Take a shoulder-width grip on a heavy barbell, your palms toward your legs. Place your feet at about shoulder width so your shins are lightly touching the bar. Straighten your arms and keep them straight throughout the movement. Flatten your back and bend your knees to dip your hips below the level of your shoulders. In the correct starting position, your hips should be above the level of your knees, and your shoulders above the level of your hips.

Starting Position

Slowly begin to straighten your legs to lift the barbell directly up from the floor. As soon as your legs are almost straight, begin to straighten your back until you are standing perfectly erect with the weight across your upper thights. Pull your shoulders back at the top of the movement. Lower the barbell back to the floor by reversing the procedure you used to raise it. Repeat the movement for the required number of repetitions.

Movement Performance

For a longer range of motion, stand on a thick block of wood (about 4 × 4 inches is good) as you do the movement.

Exercise Variations

Start.

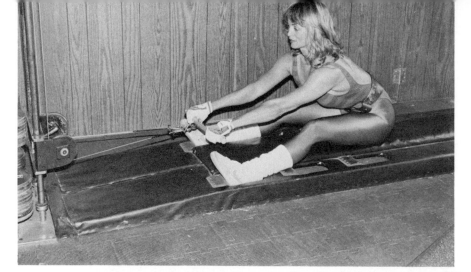

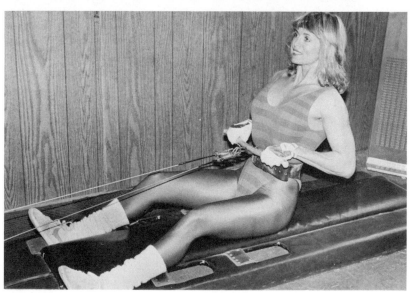

Finish.

SEATED PULLEY ROWING
Exercise Emphasis

This is one of the best of all back exercises. It builds both width and thickness in the latissimus dorsi muscles, and it places strong stress on the erector spinae and trapezius muscles.

Starting Position

Attach a handle with parallel grips to the end of a floor pulley cable. Grasp the handles with your palms facing each other. Place your feet against the foot bars of the machine, and sit back on the padded surface of the bench. Bend your legs slightly to take potential strain off your lower back, and keep them bent throughout the movement. Straighten your arms fully, and incline your torso forward toward your feet to stretch your latissimus dorsi muscles fully.

Movement Performance

Sit erect and simultaneously pull the handle of the machine slowly in to touch the lower edge of your rib cage. Hold your elbows in tight against your torso as you pull the handle in to touch your torso. Be sure to arch your back in the finish position of the movement. Slowly allow the handle and your body to return to the starting point, and repeat the movement for an appropriate number of reps.

Exercise Variations

This exercise can be done with a short, straight bar handle, a handle with shoulder-width parallel grips, or with two individual handles attached to the cable.

All bent rowing movements build latissimus dorsi thickness. Secondary emphasis is placed on the biceps, the forearm muscles, the front portion of the deltoids, and the trapezius muscles.

Stand with your left side to a flat exercise bench, bend over until your torso is parallel to the floor, and place your left hand on the bench to brace your torso in this position throughout the movement. Place your left foot forward about two feet and bend it slightly. Extend your right leg to the rear and keep it straight during the movement. Grasp a moderately heavy dumbbell in your right hand, straighten your arm completely, and rotate your right shoulder a bit toward the floor to stretch your right latissimus dorsi.

Starting Position

With your hand held so your palm is facing the midline of your body, pull the dumbbell up until it touches the side of your rib cage. Rotate your right shoulder slightly upward at the top of the movement. Slowly lower the dumbbell back to the starting point of the exercise, and repeat the movement for an appropriate number of repetitions. Be sure to do the same number of sets and repetitions for each side of your body.

Movement Performance

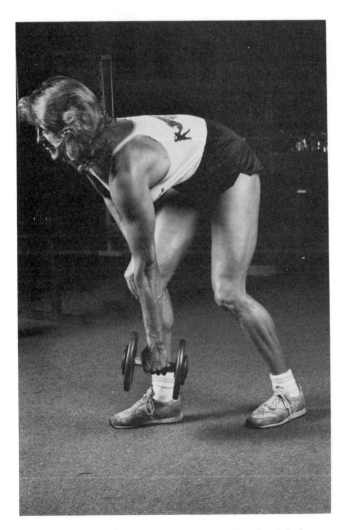 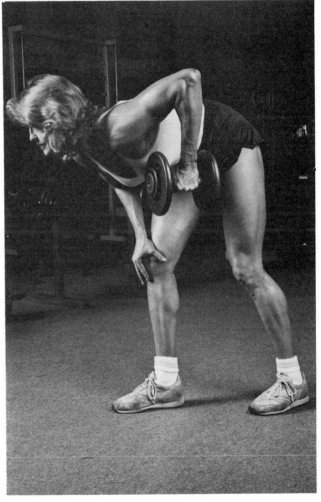

Start, working left arm with right arm braced on the right knee.   Finish.   **127**

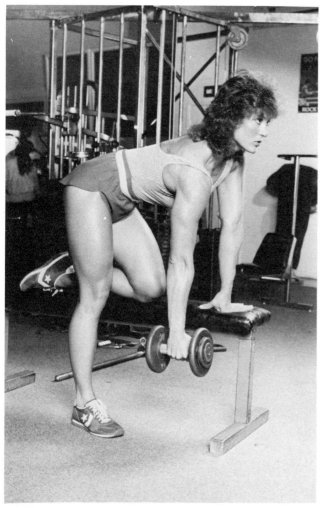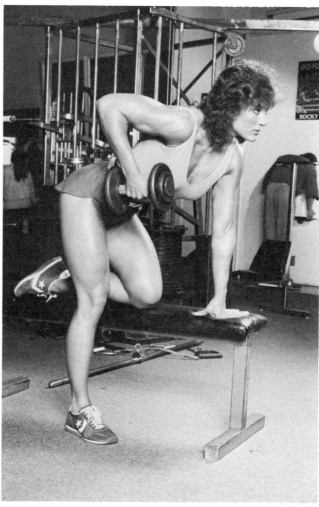

Lori Bowen demonstrates dumbbell bent rowing using bench-support alternative. This is the start.

Finish.

Exercise Variations	Many bodybuilders use an alternative leg position when doing dumbbell bent rows. Rather than placing your left foot forward as in the preceding starting position description, you can kneel with your left knee on the bench throughout the movement.
CHINS *Exercise Emphasis*	Chins develop width in the latissimus dorsi muscles. Chins done with your body pulled up so the bar touches behind your neck stress primarily the upper lats, while chins to the front of your neck stress the lower lats. Secondary stress is placed on the biceps, brachialis, and forearm muscles.
Starting Position	Take a grip on the chinning bar, with your hands set slightly wider on each side than your shoulders, your palms facing forward. Straighten your arms fully, bend your legs at right angles, and cross your ankles.
Movement Performance	Maintaining a slight arch in your back, slowly bend your arms to pull your body upward until you touch either your upper chest or trapezius muscles to the bar. Lower back to the starting point of the movement, and repeat it for the required number of repetitions.

Chins can be done with a reversed grip (your palms facing in the opposite direction) and with varying grip widths, from the hands touching each other on the bar to a position in which your hands are set as much as two feet wider than your shoulders on each side. At first you will not have enough strength in your lats and arms to do chins, and you will need to do lat pull-downs for a few weeks to develop that power. Ultimately you will be able to do chins quite easily, at which point you should add weight to your body by hanging a light dumbbell around your waist with a loop of rope.

Exercise Variations

Start, using Nautilus machine, which allows a lateral grip.

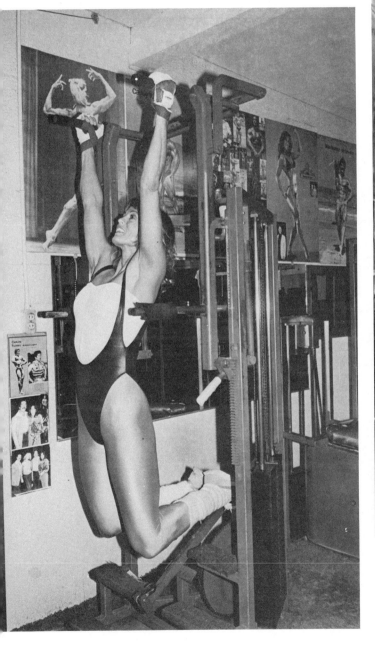

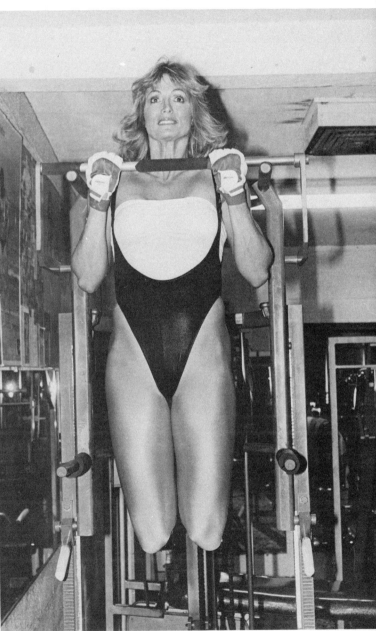

...as well as a conventional grip. (This shows the finish.)

SHOULDER EXERCISES

PRESS BEHIND THE NECK
Exercise Emphasis

Presses behind the neck strongly stress the frontal deltoids and the triceps. Secondary stress is placed on the middle and back portions of the delts and on the upper back muscles.

Starting Position

Take an overgrip on a barbell, with your hands set about four inches apart. Clean the bar to your shoulders, and push it upward to rest across your trapezius muscles behind your neck. Stand erect and tense your back muscles to maintain this position.

Movement Performance

Push the barbell directly upward until your arms are locked straight. Lower the bar back to the starting point, and repeat the movement for an appropriate number of repetitions.

Exercise Variations

You can use a wider grip when you do presses behind the neck, and you can do the movement seated to isolate your legs from the exercise.

Start.

Finish.

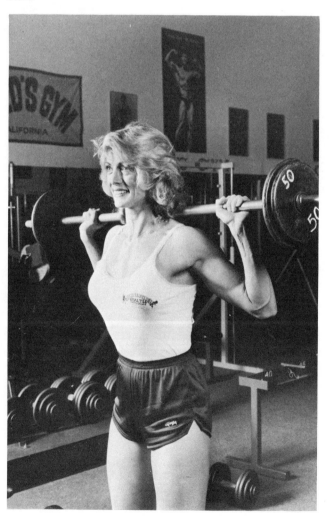
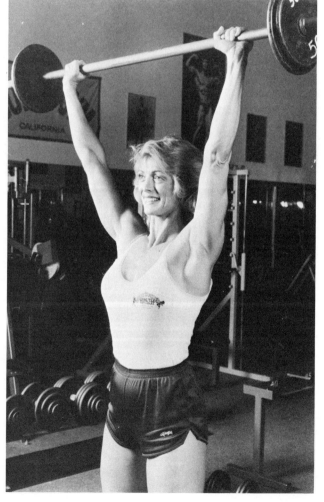

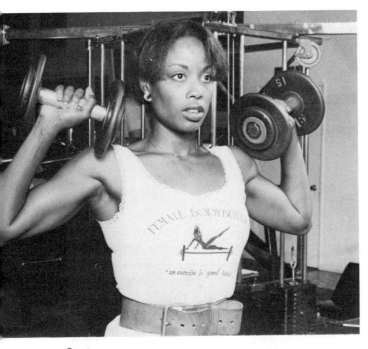

Start.

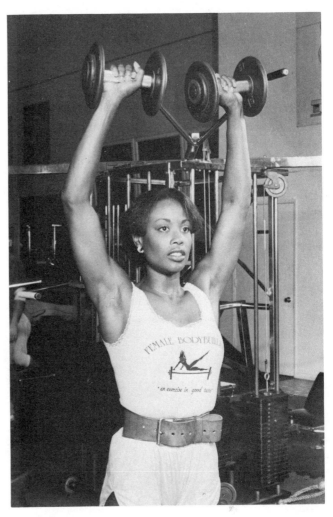

Finish.

Exercise Emphasis

This movement strongly stresses the front portion of the deltoids and the triceps. Secondary stress is placed on the rest of the delts, on the upper back, and on the upper chest muscles.

Starting Position

Clean a pair of moderately weighted dumbbells to your shoulders, and stand erect. Rotate your hands so your palms are held forward throughout the movement.

Movement Performance

Slowly push the dumbbells directly upward until they touch each other at arm's length above your head. Lower the dumbbells back to the starting point, and repeat the movement for an appropriate number of repetitions.

Exercise Variations

Rather than holding your hands with your palms forward during the movement, you can do dumbbell presses with your palms toward each other. You can also do dumbbell presses with one arm at a time while holding a solid upright with your free hand, or in alternating fashion (one dumbbell coming down as the other is pressed upward).

131

SEATED PRESSES *Exercise Emphasis*	All forms of seated presses strongly stress the deltoids at the front and the triceps. Secondary stress is placed on the rest of the deltoids and on the upper back and upper chest muscles.
Free-Weight *Starting Position*	Assume the same starting position as for military presses, presses behind the neck, or dumbbell presses, then sit at the end of a flat exercise bench and wrap your legs around the bench uprights to restrain your body in position during the movement.
Nautilus Starting *Position*	Adjust the seat of the double shoulder machine to a height that allows you to grasp the pressing handles at shoulder level. Sit in the seat and secure the lap belt around your hips. Cross your ankles and grasp the pressing handles with your palms facing each other.

Nautilus starting position.

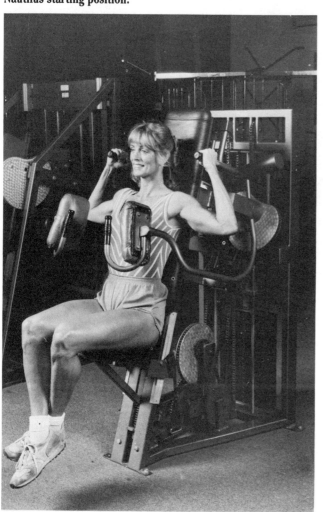

Nautilus finish.

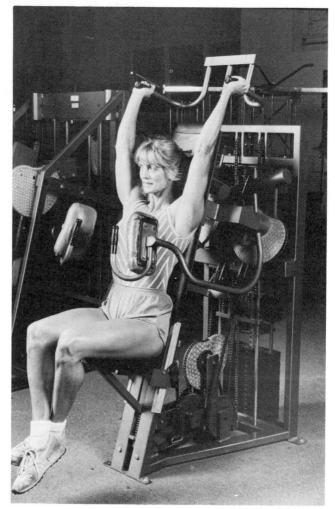

132

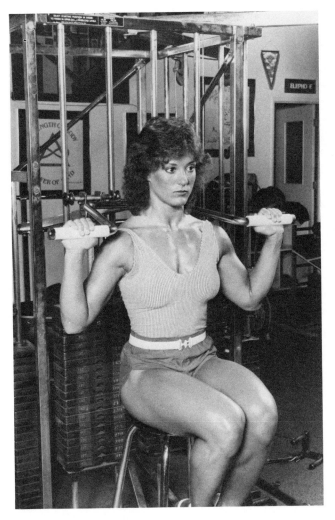

Universal starting position.

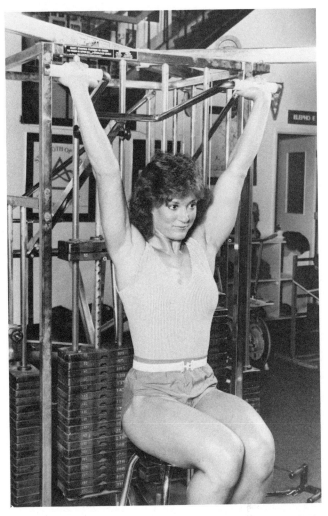

Universal finish.

Place a stool directly beneath the pressing handles of the machine, and sit on the bench either facing the machine or facing away from it. Secure your legs around the legs of the stool to restrain your body in position during the movement. Grasp the middle of the pressing handles, and sit erect on the stool.

Universal Gyms Starting Position

Slowly straighten your arms to push the handles or weight(s) to straight arm's length overhead. Lower your hands back to the starting position and repeat the movement.

Movement Performance

On all but the Nautilus machine, you can experiment with different grip widths and/or hand positions.

Exercise Variations

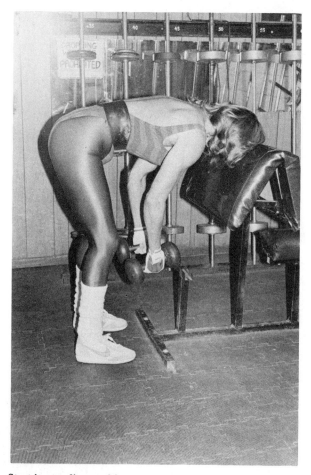

Start in standing position.

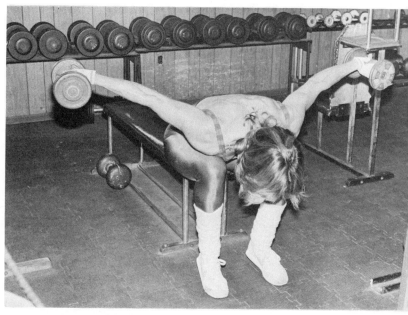

Finish, using seated position.

BENT LATERALS *Exercise Emphasis*	Bent laterals place primary stress on the back portion of the deltoids and secondary stress on the upper back muscles.
Starting Position	Place your feet at shoulder width, grasp two light dumbbells, and bend forward at the waist until your torso is parallel to the floor. Hang your arms directly down from your shoulders, with your palms toward each other and the dumbbells touching directly beneath the center of your chest. Bend your arms slightly.
Movement Performance	Slowly raise the dumbbells in semicircular arcs directly out to the sides until they are slightly above the level of your shoulders. Lower the weights back to the starting point of the exercise, and repeat the movement for an appropriate number of repetitions.
Exercise Variations	You can do bent laterals using two dumbbells while seated at the end of a flat exercise bench, with your torso resting on your thighs. Another common variation is done with cables providing the resistance.

ARM EXERCISES

Nautilus curls strongly stress the biceps muscles and place minor secondary stress on the flexor muscles of the forearms.

NAUTILUS CURLS
Exercise Emphasis

Adjust the seat height until it is set in a position so your shoulders are slightly below the bottom edge of the angled pad of the machine. Grasp the movable handles with your palms upward, and sit down in the machine's seat. Fully straighten your arms.

Starting Position

Keeping your right arm straight, slowly bend your left arm as fully as possible. Return your left arm to the starting position, and do the next repetition with your right arm. Alternate arms until you have done the required number of repetitions with each one.

Movement Performance

For a better peak contraction effect, you can curl both handles to your shoulders and hold this position with one arm while the other is straightened and then bent again. You can do Nautilus curls with one arm at a time.

Exercise Variations

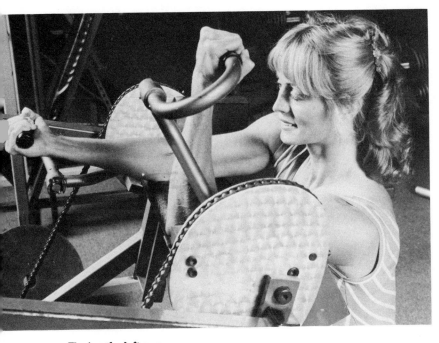

Flexing the left arm.

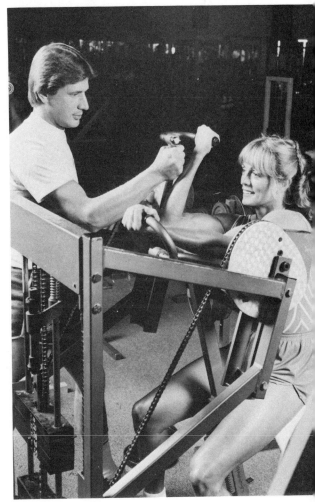

A forced rep.

| *PULLEY CURLS* | This exercise strongly stresses the biceps muscles and places minor secondary stress on |
| *Exercise Emphasis* | the flexor muscles of the forearms. |

PULLEY CURLS
Exercise Emphasis   This exercise strongly stresses the biceps muscles and places minor secondary stress on the flexor muscles of the forearms.

Starting Position   Attach a straight bar handle to the cable running through a floor pulley. Grasp the handle with an undergrip, and stand back about two feet from the pulley. Press your upper arms aginst the sides of your torso, and keep them in this position throughout the movement. Straighten your arms fully.

Movement Performance   Slowly bend your arms fully to move the cable handle in a semicircle from a position in front of your thighs to one just beneath your chin. Return your arms to the starting position of the exercise, and repeat the movement for the required number of repetitions.

Exercise Variations   You can do this movement with an overgrip, which stresses the brachialis and forearm muscles. You can also do pulley curls with one hand grasping a loop handle attached to the cable and the elbow of your working arm pressed into the side of your waist.

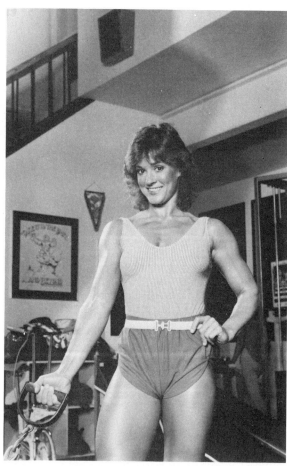

Start.

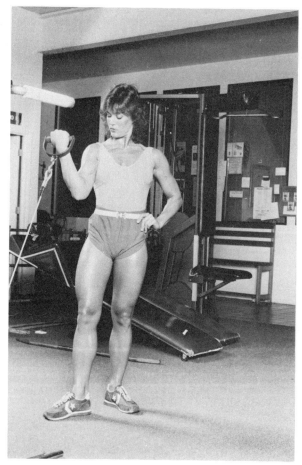

Finish.

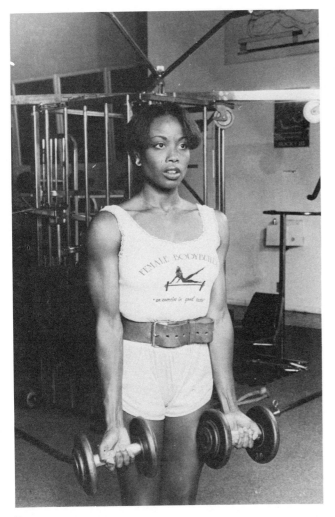

Start.

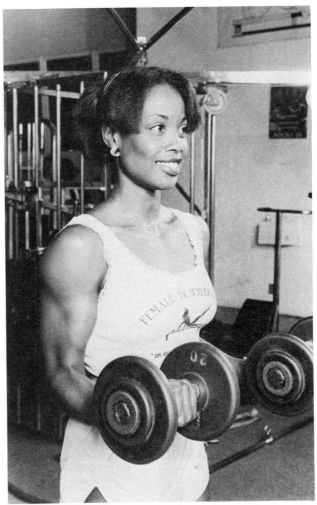

Finish.

Dumbbell curls strongly stress the biceps muscles. Secondary stress is placed on the flexor muscles of the forearms.

DUMBBELL CURLS
Exercise Emphasis

Grasp two moderately weighted dumbbells, and stand erect with your arms hanging down at your sides. Your palms should be facing each other. Press your upper arms against the sides of your torso, and keep them in this position throughout the movement.

Starting Position

Simultaneously curl the dumbbells up to your shoulders, and rotate your hands so your palms are facing upward at the top of the movement. Lower the dumbbells back to the starting point, and repeat the movement for an appropriate number of reps.

Movement Performance

You can do dumbbell curls alternately, one dumbbell descending as the other is curled upward. Normal and alternate dumbbell curls can both be done while seated at the end of a flat exercise bench.

Exercise Variations

137

LYING BARBELL TRICEPS EXTENSIONS
Exercise Emphasis

This movement isolates stress on the triceps muscles.

Starting Position

Take a narrow overgrip in the middle of a barbell (there should be four to six inches of space between your hands on the bar). Lie back on a flat exercise bench and extend your arms directly upward.

Movement Performance

Keeping your upper arms motionless, bend your elbows and allow the barbell to travel in a semicircular arc from the starting point until it touches your forehead. Use your triceps strength to return the barbell back along the same arc to the starting point, and repeat the movement.

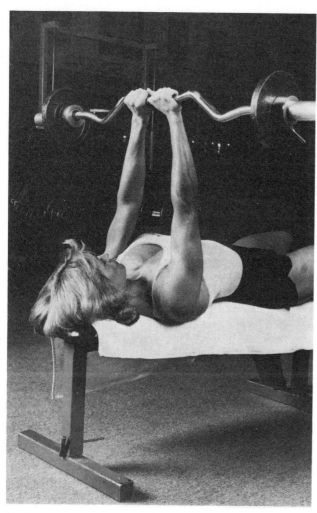

Start.

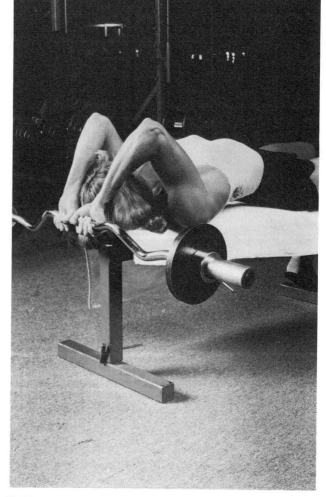

Finish.

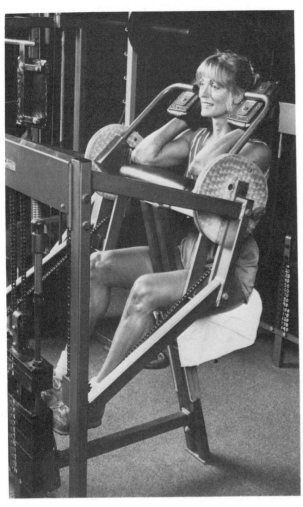

Start.

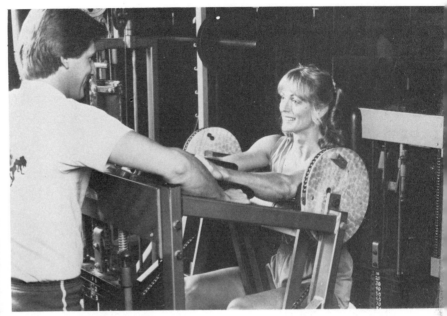

Finish.

Nautilus triceps extensions isolate stress on the triceps muscles.

Adjust the seat so that your shoulders are slightly below the bottom edge of the angled pad of the machine when you are seated. With your palms facing each other, place the edges of your hands against the movable pads of the machine. Bend your arms fully.

Starting Position

Slowly extend your arms. Return your arms to the starting position, and repeat the movement for an appropriate number of reps.

Movement Performance

For a better peak contraction effect, you can extend both arms and hold that position with one arm while the other is bent and then straightened again.

Exercise Variations

**BARBELL REVERSE
CURLS
Exercise Emphasis**   All forms of reverse curls stress the biceps, brachialis, and forearm muscles.

Starting Position   Take a shoulder-width overgrip on a barbell. Stand erect with the bar resting across your upper thighs and your upper arms against the sides of your torso.

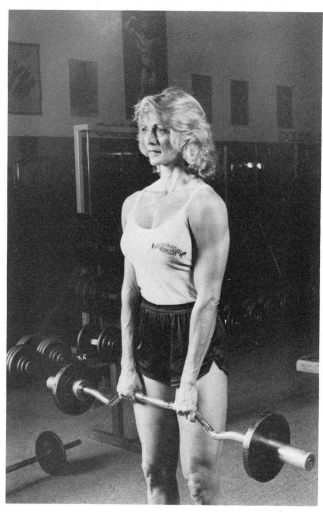

Start.

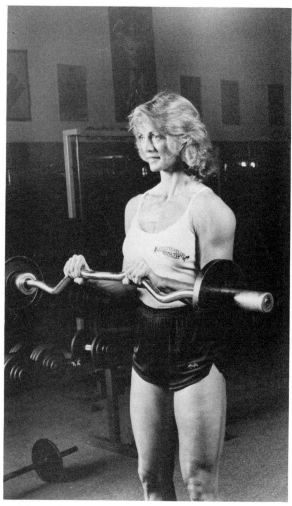

Finish.

Movement Performance   Slowly bend your arms to curl the barbell up to your chin. Lower the weight back to the starting position, and repeat the movement for the desired number of repetitions.

Exercise Variations   You can do this movement with a more narrow grip.

Done with your palms up, dumbbell wrist curls stress the powerful flexor muscles of your forearms. Performed with your palms down, the exercise stresses the smaller extensor muscles of your forearms.

Grasp two moderately weighted dumbbells, sit at the end of a flat exercise bench, and run your forearms down your thighs so that your fists are off the edge of your knees. Sag your fists downward as far as possible, palms up or down.

Curl the weight upward as high as possible by fully flexing your wrists. Lower the bar back to the starting point of the movement, and repeat it for an appropriate number of repetitions.

This exercise can be done one arm at a time, with your forearm running across the surface of a padded exercise bench.

DUMBBELL WRIST CURLS
Exercise Emphasis

Starting Position

Movement Performance

Exercise Variations

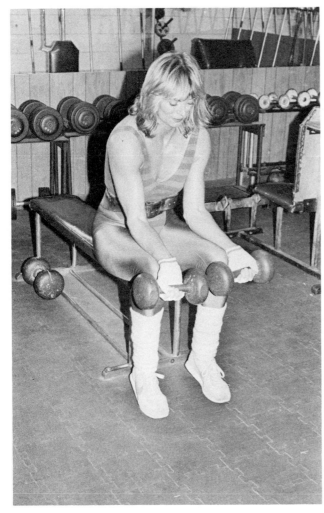

Start.

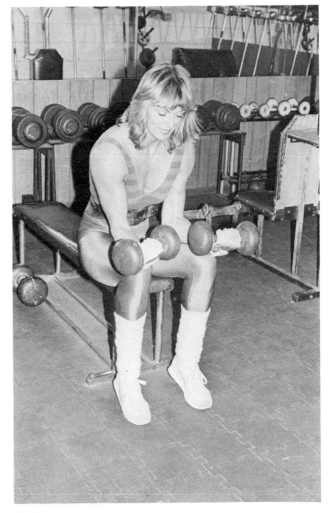

Finish.

141

CALF EXERCISES

CALF PRESSES
Exercise Emphasis
Calf presses can be done on a vertical leg press machine, angled leg press machine, Nautilus leg press machine, or Universal Gyms leg press machine. All four directly stress the large gastrocnemius muscles of the calves.

Starting Position
Regardless of the machine used, sit or lie in it, place your feet on the platform or pedals, and extend your legs completely. Then slide all of your feet but your toes and the balls off the edge of the platform or pedals. Relax your calves and allow your toes to move as far toward your face as possible.

Start, using vertical leg press machine.

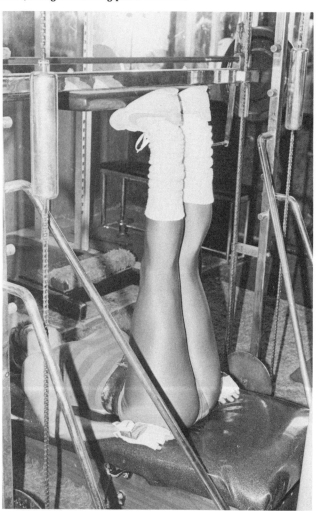

Finish, calves flexed.

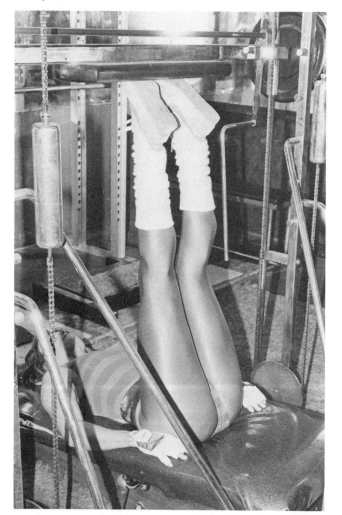

142

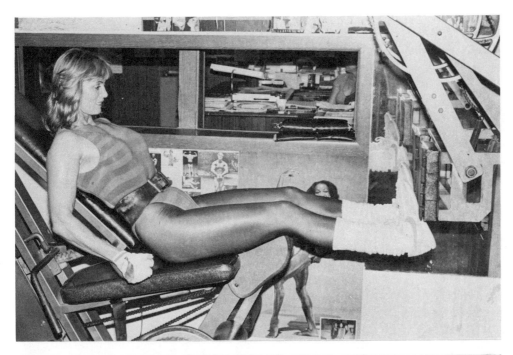

Nautilus start.

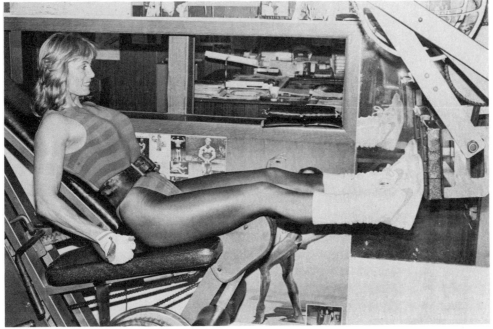

Nautilus finish.

Slowly extend your feet as far as you can. Allow the weight to push your toes back to the starting point and repeat the movement.

Movement Performance

Be sure to alternate between the three foot angles used on all calf exercises (toes straight ahead, angled inward, and angled outward). On the two free-weight machines, you can also vary the width of your foot placement on the movable platform.

Exercise Variations

143

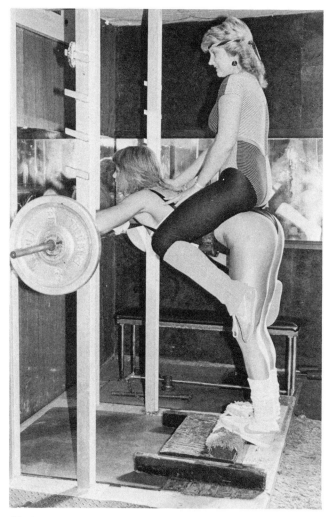 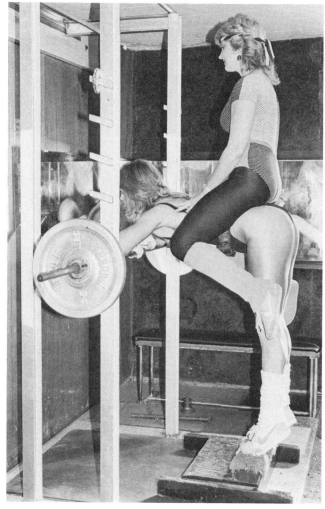

Start.   Finish.

DONKEY CALF RAISES
Exercise Emphasis

This is usually an amusing movement to see performed, but it is one of the best gastrocnemius exercises.

Starting Position

Place a toe block about two feet from the end of a flat exercise bench. Step on the toe block with your feet about ten inches apart, your toes pointed straight ahead, and only the toes and balls of your feet on the block. Bend at the waist, and place your hands on the bench to keep your torso parallel to the floor during the movement. Have a heavy training partner jump up astride your hips and balance himself/herself in position by grasping the sides of your torso. Relax your calves and allow your heels to sink as far below the level of your toes as possible.

Movement Performance

Slowly rise up on your toes to the limit of your ankle range of motion. Sink back to the starting point, and repeat the movement for an appropriate number of repetitions.

Exercise Variations

Be sure to use the standard three toe positions, and vary the width of your toe placement from time to time. If your training partner is too light, he or she can hold an additional barbell plate against the small of your back as you do the movement.

144

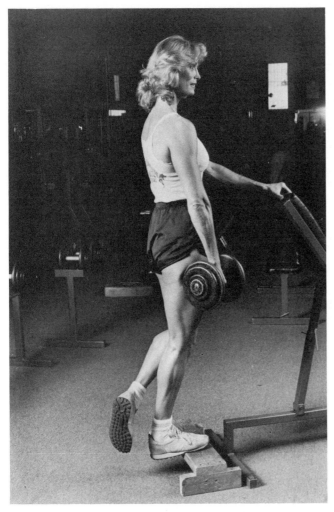

Start.

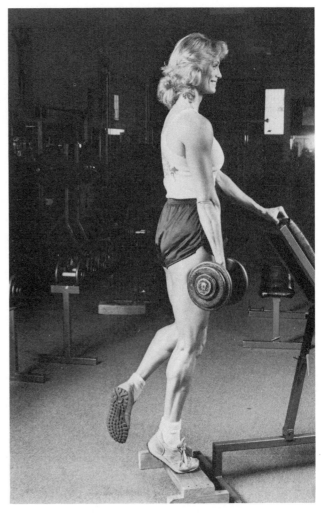

Finish.

This simple calf movement can be done with no equipment other than a dumbbell and a block of wood. One-legged toe raises directly stress the gastrocnemius muscles.

ONE-LEGGED TOE RAISES
Exercise Emphasis

Place the toes and ball of your left foot on either a block of wood or a stair riser. Grasp a moderately weighted dumbbell in your left hand, bend your right leg at a 90-degree angle to keep it out of the movement, and grasp a sturdy upright with your right hand to balance your body during the movement. Sag your left heel as far below the level of your toes as possible.

Starting Position

Slowly rise up as high as you can on the toes of your left foot, lower your body back to the starting point of the exercise, and repeat the movement for the required number of repetitions. Switch feet.

Movement Performance

It is a bit difficult to angle your foot inward as you do this exercise, but you can use the toes-ahead and toes-out foot positions quite easily. By pulling up slightly with your balancing hand, you can give yourself a few forced reps (i.e., you can force your calf muscles to keep working past the point where they would normally fail).

Exercise Variations

145

MIDSECTION EXERCISES

NAUTILUS CRUNCHES *Exercise Emphasis*	All forms of crunches—and particularly those done on an abdominal machine—strongly stress the frontal abdominal muscles.
Starting Position	Adjust the height of the seat to a position where the movable handles are a bit above shoulder level when you sit in the seat. Sit down in the machine, hook your insteps beneath the roller pad, and grasp the handles near your shoulders. Allow the machine to stretch your frontal torso muscles by pulling upward on your hands and shoulders.
Movement Performance	Force your shoulders toward your hips by crunching your torso and leaning slightly forward under resistance. Return to the starting point of the exercise, and repeat it for the desired number of repetitions.
Exercise Variations	For a more intense stimulation of your abdominal muscles, try to hold the bottom position of this movement for a slow count of two before allowing the weight to pull your body back to the starting position. You can also stress the intercostal muscles to a degree by twisting slightly to each side on alternate reps as you crunch down in the exercise.

Start.

Finish.

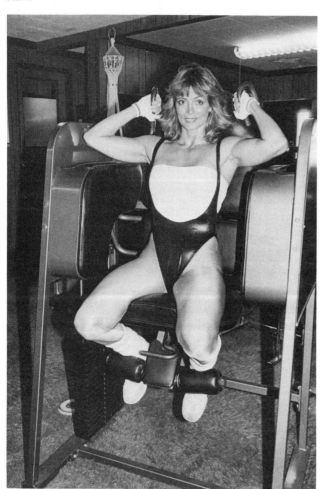
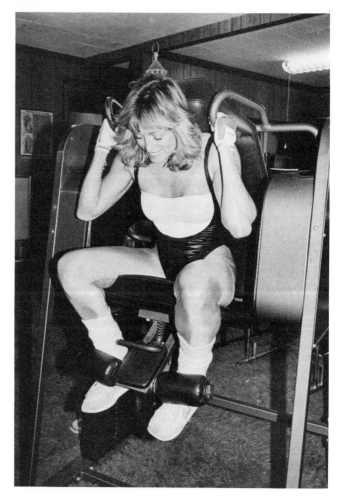

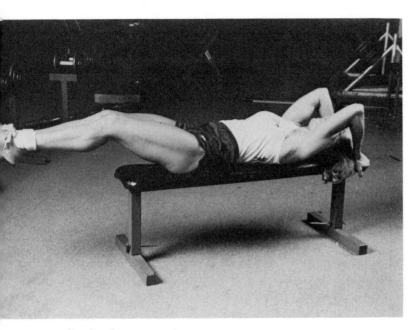

Starting the movement.

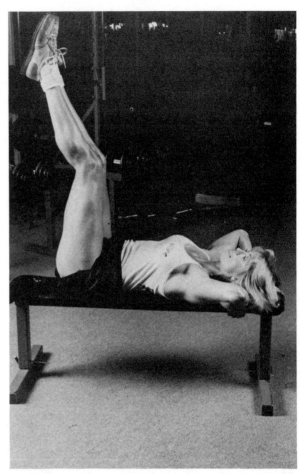

Finish.

Bench leg raises stress the entire frontal abdominal wall, particularly the lower half of the rectus abdominis muscle group.

BENCH LEG RAISES
Exercise Emphasis

Lie on your back on a flat exercise bench, with your buttocks at one end of the bench. Reach behind your head and grasp the edges of the bench with your hands to restrain your torso in position on the bench during the exercise. Bend your legs slightly to keep undue strain off your lower back, and keep them bent throughout the movement. Lower your feet to a position near the floor.

Starting Position

Slowly raise your feet in a semicircular arc from the starting point to a position directly above your hips. Lower your feet back along the same arc to the starting point, and repeat the movement for an appropriate number of repetitions.

Movement Performance

The higher the bench you use for these leg raises, the greater the stretch you can feel in your abdominal muscles. Some bodybuilders prefer to do bench leg raises with their ankles crossed. If this movement becomes easy to do, you can add resistance to it by holding a light dumbbell between your feet.

Exercise Variations

147

CRUNCHES Exercise Emphasis	All forms of crunches stress the rectus abdominis muscle group, particularly the upper half of the abdominal wall.
Starting Position	Lie on your back on the floor with your calves draped over a flat exercise bench so that your thighs are perpendicular to the floor. Place your hands behind your head during the exercise.
Movement Performance	You must simultaneously do four things to perform this movement: (1) raise your hips from the floor with lower abdominal strength; (2) raise your shoulders from the floor with upper abdominal strength; (3) force your shoulders toward your hips; and (4) exhale sharply. If you adhere to form, you will feel a strong contraction in your abdominal muscles at the top of the movement. Relax your abdominal muscles to return your body to the starting point, and repeat the movement for the required number of repetitions.
Exercise Variations	There are two alternate starting positions that can be used for crunches. In the first, you lie on your back on the floor with your legs running straight up a wall and your hips in the angle formed by the floor and wall. In this position, you won't be able to lift your hips from the floor, but you will nonetheless feel a strong contraction in your abdominals. Second, you can largely duplicate the usual starting position by lying on your back with your hips about eighteen inches from the wall and your feet flat on the wall at knee level. Regardless of the variation used, you can involve the intercostal muscles by twisting alternately to each side as you do the movement.

Start.

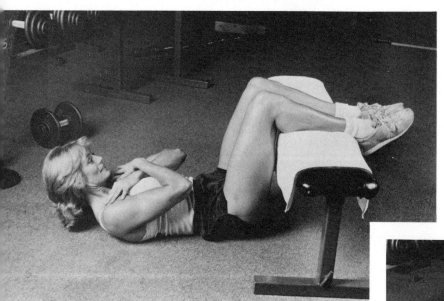

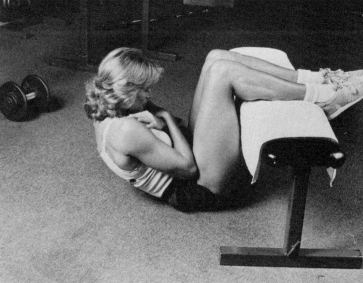

148   **Finish.**

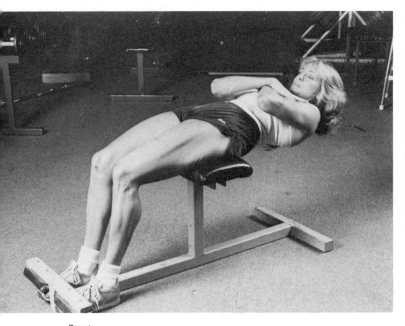

Start.

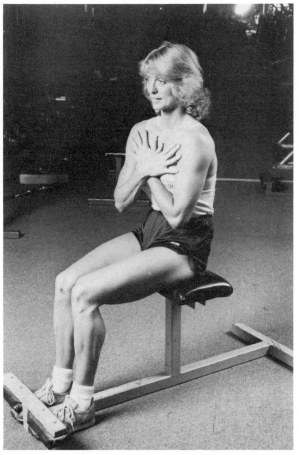

Finish.

This popular short-range movement is performed to stress the rectus abdominis muscles, particularly the upper half of the frontal abdominal wall.

Sit on the seat of a Roman chair, and hook your toes under the bar of the bench. Cross your arms over your chest, and lean back until your torso is at less than a 45-degree angle to the floor.

Starting Position

Sit forward until you begin to feel stress coming off your abdominals, a position a few degrees short of having your torso perfectly upright. Rock back and forth between these two torso positions for the desired number of repetitions.

Movement Performance

You can stress the intercostals by twisting alternately to each side as you do the exercise. With both this variation and the normal straight Roman chair sit-ups, you can add resistance by holding a light barbell plate over your chest.

Exercise Variations

149

LEVEL TWO WORKOUTS

As with Level One Workouts, you can follow each of the three training programs presented in this section for four to six weeks before progressing to the next level of intensity. By now you will have determined how your temperament affects the length of time you spend on a particular routine, and you will know how soon to switch to a new workout.

Remember while following these training schedules that *the greater the intensity of each set for a particular muscle group, the less total sets you can perform for that muscle.* The first two routines in this section are meant to condition your body further to the stress of high-intensity training, so you will do more and more total sets for each muscle group in the first and second programs. With the third routine in this section, however, you will begin to follow high-intensity training techniques, and that will reduce the total number of sets you perform for each body part.

The trend toward doing less sets will continue through the Level Three Workouts in the next chapter, until you are performing only a few more sets for each muscle group than you did in the second Level One Workout.

FIRST LEVEL TWO WORKOUT   With this workout, you will begin to use a four-day split routine. A split routine will allow you to do two workouts each week for your major muscle groups.

MONDAY/THURSDAY

Exercise	Sets	Reps
1. Roman chair sit-ups	2	20–30
2. Bench leg raises	2	20–30
3. Seated twisting	2	50
4. Incline dumbbell presses	3	6–10
5. Pec deck flyes	2	8–12
6. Decline barbell presses	2	6–10
7. Seated dumbbell presses	3	6–10
8. Side laterals	2	8–12
9. Bent laterals	2	8–12
10. Lying barbell triceps extensions	3	8–12
11. Pulley push-downs	2	8–12
12. Dumbbell wrist curls	4	10–15
13. Donkey calf raises	3	10–15
14. Seated calf raises	3	10–15

TUESDAY/FRIDAY

Exercise	Sets	Reps
1. Crunches	2	20–30
2. Leg raises	2	20–30
3. Seated twists	2	50
4. Leg presses	4	10–15
5. Hack squats	3	10–15
6. Leg curls	4	10–15
7. Cable leg adductions	3	10–15
8. Deadlifts	2	6–8
9. Chins	3	8–12
10. Seated pulley rowing	3	8–12
11. Barbell shrugs	3	10–15
12. Dumbbell curls	3	8–12
13. Barbell reverse curls	3	8–12
14. Barbell wrist curls	3	10–15
15. Calf presses	5	10–15

SECOND LEVEL TWO WORKOUT

This split routine is the final one in which you will increase training intensity by adding to the number of sets you perform for each muscle group. Past this level, you will increase intensity by training harder within each set. And when you increase intraset training intensity, you will actually be forced to reduce the number of sets you do for each body part.

MONDAY/THURSDAY

Exercise	Sets	Reps
1. Nautilus crunches	2–3	10–20
2. Incline leg raises	2–3	20–30
3. Seated twisting	2–3	50
4. Incline barbell presses	3	6-10
5. Parallel bar dips	3	6-10
6. Flat-bench flyes	2	8–12
7. Seated presses behind the neck	3	6-10
8. One-arm dumbbell side laterals	3	8–12
9. Seated bent laterals	3	8–12
10. Nautilus triceps extensions	3	8–12
11. Pulley push-downs	2	8–12
12. Dumbbell wrist curls	3	10–15
13. Barbell reverse wrist curls	3	10–15
14. Standing calf raises	3–4	10–15
15. One-legged calf raises	3–4	10–15

TUESDAY/FRIDAY

Exercise	Sets	Reps
1. Incline sit-ups	2–3	20–30
2. Bench leg raises	2–3	20–30
3. Seated twist	2–3	20–30
4. Hyperextensions	3	10–15
5. Seated pulley rowing	3	8–12
6. Dumbbell bent rowing	3	8–12
7. Lat pull-downs	2	8–12
8. Upright rowing	3	8–12
9. Nautilus hip and back	2	10–15
10. Cable abductions	2	10–15
11. Cable adductions	2	10–15
12. Squats	3	10–15
13. Leg extensions	3	10–15
14. Leg curls	4	10–15
15. Nautilus curls	4	8–12
16. Barbell reverse curls	3	8–12
17. Barbell wrist curls	3	10–15
18. Donkey calf raises	4–5	10–15

THIRD LEVEL TWO WORKOUT

With this routine, you will use forced reps for the final set of each recommended exercise. (Review Chapter 4 to refresh your understanding of advanced training techniques.) You will need a training partner to perform forced reps. She or he will pull up on the barbell, machine, or dumbbells just enough to allow you to complete two or three forced reps past the point at which your muscles would ordinarily be too fatigued to complete more repetitions. You won't need more than two or three forced reps on each exercise at this point to increase your training intensity markedly. And you needn't do forced reps for your abdominal muscles.

MONDAY/THURSDAY

Exercise	Sets	Reps
1. Twisting incline sit-ups	3	20–30
2. Bench leg raises	3	20–30
3. Seated twists	3	50
4. Incline dumbbell presses	2	6–10
5. Decline barbell presses	2	6–10
6. Pec deck flyes	2	8–12
7. Seated dumbbell presses	2	6–10
8. Nautilus side laterals	2	8–12
9. Bent laterals	2	8–12
10. Upright rowing	2	8–12
11. Chins behind the neck	2	8–12
12. Seated pulley rowing	2	8–12
13. Front lat pull-downs	2	8–12
14. Barbell reverse curls	2	8–12
15. Barbell wrist curls	2	10–15
16. Seated calf raises	2	8–10
17. Calf presses	1	10–12
18. Donkey calf raises	1	12–15

TUESDAY/FRIDAY

Exercise	Sets	Reps
1. Nautilus crunches	3	10–20
2. Wall crunches	3	20–30
3. Seated twisting	3	50
4. Deadlifts	3	6–8
5. Leg presses	3	10–15
6. Leg extensions	2	10–15
7. Leg curls	3	10–15
8. Lunges	1–2	10–15
9. Seated dumbbell curls	2	8–12
10. Nautilus curls	2	8–12
11. Nautilus triceps extensions	2	8–12
12. Lying barbell triceps extensions	2	8–12
13. Dumbbell wrist curls	2	10–15
14. Barbell reverse wrist curls	2	10–15
15. Standing calf raises	2	10–15
16. One-legged calf raises	2	10–15

LEVEL THREE WORKOUTS | 8

In this advanced exercise and workout chapter, I will present more than thirty new exercises but only one training program. By now you will already know how to make up your own routines, and you no doubt already have a good feel for how your body responds to various training techniques. Once you have developed an instinctive sense for the effect training and diet have on your body, you should always formulate your own routines rather than following those you find in weight training and bodybuilding books and magazines.

THIGH AND HIP EXERCISES

Partial squats can be performed with much heavier weights than used for full squats. All variations of the squat strongly stress the quadriceps, buttocks, hip, and lower back muscles. Secondary stress is placed on the hamstrings, upper back muscles, and abdominals.

PARTIAL SQUATS
Exercise Emphasis

Place a barbell on a squat rack, and load it with an appropriate poundage for a set of partial squats. Step under the bar and bend your knees so you can position the bar across your shoulders behind your neck. Grasp the bar out near the plates on each side to balance it across your shoulders, and straighten your legs to remove the bar from the rack. Step back one or two paces and position your feet at shoulder width, your toes angled slightly outward. Focus your eyes on a point at head level on the wall in front of yourself, and keep them focused on this spot throughout your set. Tense your back muscles and keep them tensed throughout the set.

Starting Position

Keeping your torso erect throughout the movement, slowly bend your knees and sink down to a position with your thighs parallel to the floor. Then fully straighten your legs. This is called a parallel squat. You can also do half squats (squatting half of the way down

Movement Performance

155

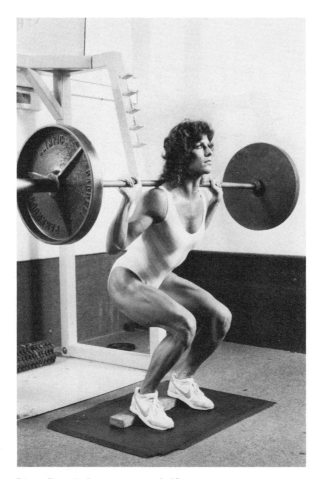

Diana Dennis demonstrates a half squat.

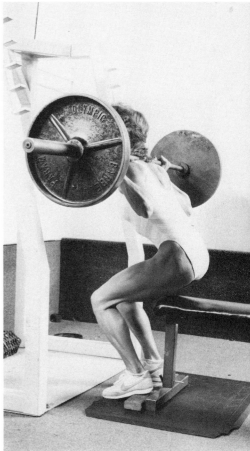

Here Diana demonstrates a bench squat.

to a full position) and quarter squats. One specialized form of squats is called bench squats. In this exercise you straddle a flat exercise bench and squat down until your buttocks lightly touch the bench before recovering to a position with your legs straight. Be sure to have two spotters available at the ends of the bar when you are doing partial squats.

Exercise Variations   Many gyms have a power rack consisting of four wood or metal uprights with holes drilled in them. You can fit steel bars through the holds in the uprights to catch the loaded bar at any level you wish. If you have a power rack available, you should use it for your partial squats.

NAUTILUS HIP
ADDUCTION/
ABDUCTION
Exercise Emphasis   When you force your thighs together using this machine, you strongly stress the adductor muscles of your inner thighs. When pushing your legs away from each other under resistance using this machine, you stress the muscles at the sides of your hips and upper/outer thighs.

Starting Position   Sit in the machine and recline against the backrest. Fasten the lap belt around your hips, and place your legs between the pads of the movement arms. A rotating level at the side of the machine allows you to select the direction from which you apply resistance, and

this should be set to the correct selection before entering the machine.

From a position with your legs completely spread apart, slowly force them closed against the resistance provided by the machine. Or, with the lever set to the opposite selection, you can force your legs apart from a position together at the start of the movement. *Movement Performance*

To achieve a better peak contraction in your working muscles, you can hold the contracted position of each repetition for a slow count of two. *Exercise Variations*

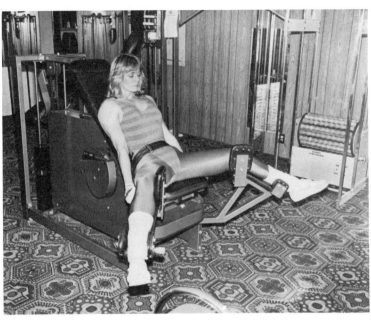

Adduction Start.

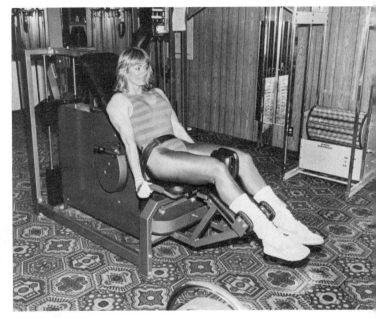

Adduction finish.

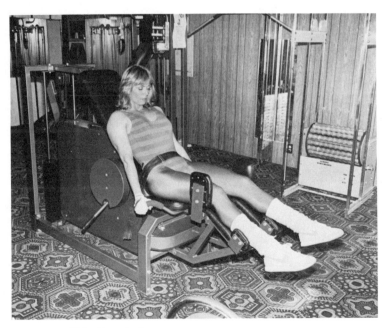

Abduction start.

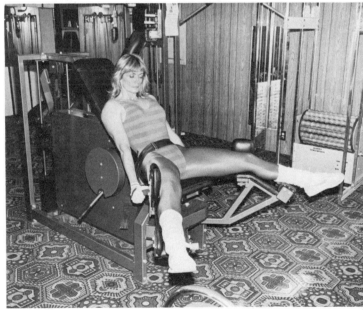

Abduction finish.

157

CHEST EXERCISES

INCLINE/DECLINE
FLYES
Exercise Emphasis

Incline flyes isolate stress on the upper pectorals and frontal deltoids. Decline flyes shift stress to the lower pecs.

Starting Position

Grasp two moderately weighted dumbbells, and lie back on an incline or decline bench. Extend your arms directly upward from your shoulder joints and perpendicular to the floor. Bend your arms slightly and keep them bent throughout the movement.

Movement Performance

Slowly lower the dumbbells directly out to the sides in semicircular arcs to as low a position below the level of your shoulders as possible. Then slowly return the dumbbells back along the same arcs to the starting point, and repeat the movement for an appropriate number of repetitions.

Exercise Variations

You can do both incline and decline flyes on a variety of inclines. It is also possible to do all forms of flyes with two floor pulleys, which keeps continuous tension on your working pectoral muscles.

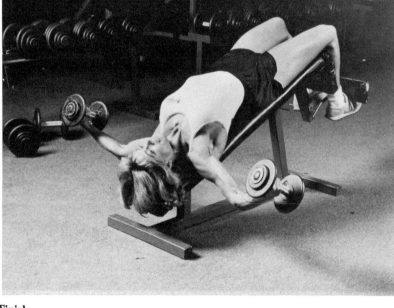

Finish.

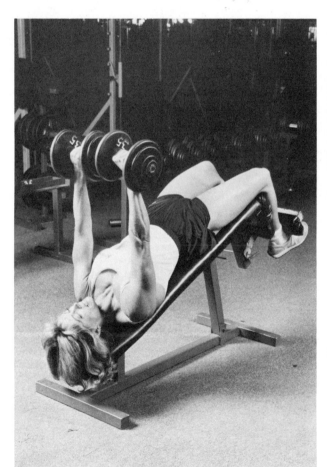

Start (decline).

158

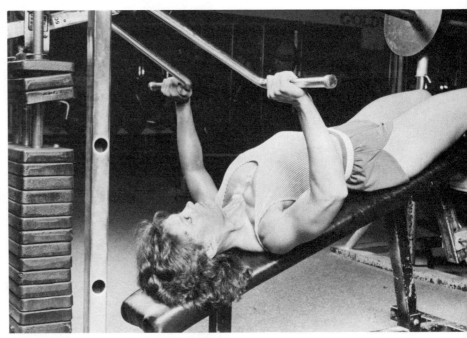

Decline press on Universal machine, midpoint.

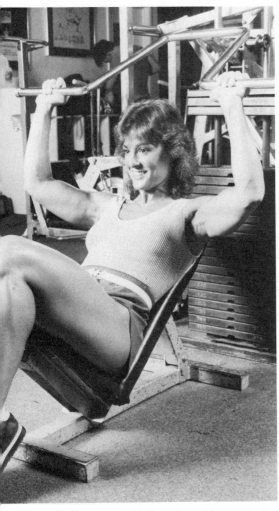

Incline press on Universal machine, midpoint.

Incline presses performed on a machine stress the upper pectorals, the front portion of the deltoids, and the triceps. Machine decline presses stress the lower pectorals and again the frontal deltoids and the triceps. Both variations of machine bench presses secondarily stress the latissimus dorsi muscles and center portion of the deltoids.

MACHINE INCLINE/ DECLINE PRESSES Exercise Emphasis

Place an incline or decline bench either beneath the bench press station of a Universal Gyms machine or under a Smith machine (one in which the weight slides up and down two uprights). Lie back on the bench and take a grip on the bar or movement handles with your hands set four or five inches wider than your shoulders on each side. Straighten your arms fully.

Starting Position

While holding your elbows directly out to the sides, slowly lower the barbell down to touch your upper chest (incline presses) or lower chest (decline presses). Push the barbell back to the starting point, and repeat the movement for the required number of repetitions.

Movement Performance

You can use various grip widths on the bar when using these two exercises, as well as various degrees of incline and decline.

Exercise Variations

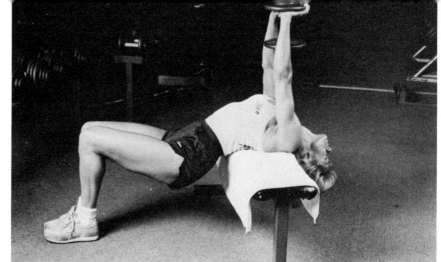

Start.

Finish.

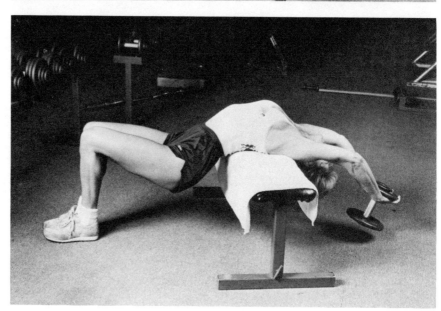

CROSS-BENCH DUMBBELL PULLOVERS
Exercise Emphasis

All forms of pullovers place primary stress on the pectorals and secondary emphasis on the latissimus dorsi muscles.

Starting Position

Place a dumbbell on end on the padded surface of an exercise bench. Rest your shoulders and upper back across the bench, and place your feet about shoulder-width apart on the floor to balance your body in position during the movement. Rest your palms under the upper plates of the dumbbell, and hook your thumbs around the dumbbell handle. Pull the dumbbell into a position at straight arm's length directly above your upper chest. Bend your arms slightly and keep them bent throughout the movement.

Movement Performance

Slowly lower the dumbbell in a semicircular arc from the starting point to a position as close to the floor behind your head as possible. Return the dumbbell back along the same arc to the starting point, and repeat the movement for the desired number of repetitions.

Exercise Variations

To achieve a greater stretch in your working muscles, you should lower your hips four to six inches as the dumbbell reaches the low point of the exercise. Dumbbell pullovers can also be done lying lengthwise on the bench with either a single dumbbell or a dumbbell in each hand.

160

This movement places primary stress on the pectorals and secondary emphasis on the latissimus dorsi muscles. Done in conjunction with deep breathing, stiff-arm pullovers also help to enlarge the rib cage.

STIFF-ARM PULLOVERS
Exercise Emphasis

Grasp a light barbell with a shoulder-width overgrip, and lie lengthwise along a flat exercise bench, your head hanging off the edge. Straighten your arms and hold the barbell directly above your shoulder joints.

Starting Position

Keeping your arms straight, slowly lower the barbell in a semicircular arc to as low a position behind your head as possible. Return the weight along the same arc to the starting position, and repeat the movement for an appropriate number of repetitions.

Movement Performance

You can vary the width of your grip on the barbell as you do the movement. You can also do a bent-arm pullover movement using a narrow grip (about six inches between your hands on the bar and with your elbows bent at 90-degree angles throughout the movement).

Exercise Variations

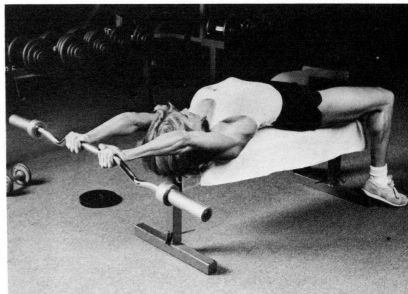

Finish.

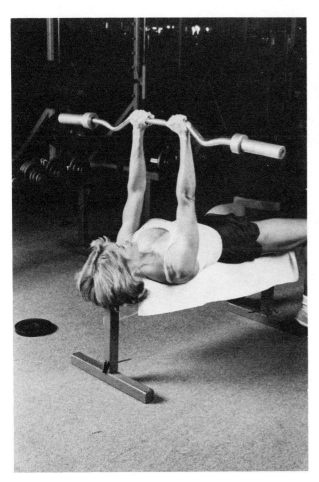

Start.

161

NAUTILUS PULLOVERS
Exercise Emphasis

Pullovers performed on a Nautilus machine strongly stress both the pectorals and latissimus dorsi muscles. Secondary stress is on the serratus, intercostal, and rectus abdominis muscles.

Starting Position

Adjust the seat of the machine so your shoulder joints are at the same level as the middle of the machine's cams on each side of your body. Sit in the seat, fasten the lap belt around your hips, push down on the foot bar to bring the movement pads into position so you can place your elbows against them, release the foot bar, and allow your arms and elbows to travel upward and backward as far as comfortably possible.

Movement Performance

Using pectoral and latissimus dorsi strength, move your elbows forward and downward as far as possible. Allow the weight to pull your elbows back to the starting position, and repeat the movement for the required number of repetitions.

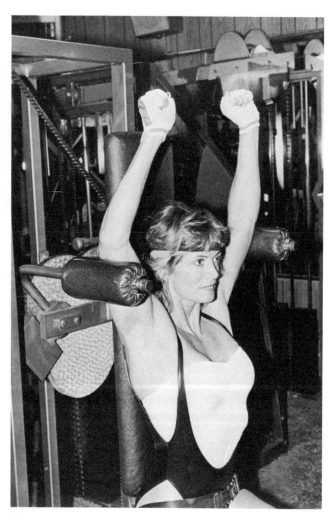

Start.

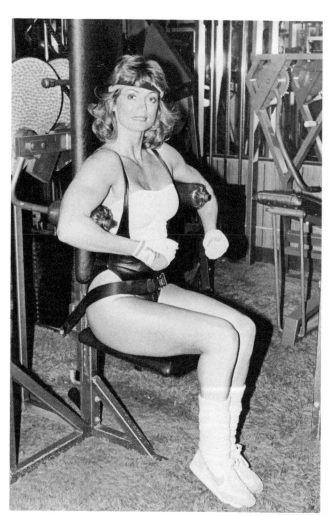

Finish.

162

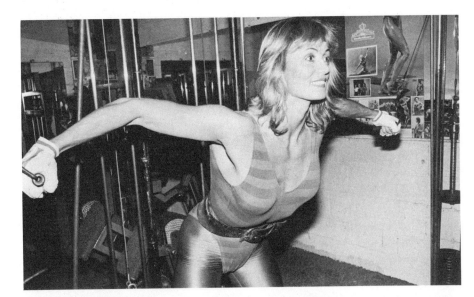

Start.

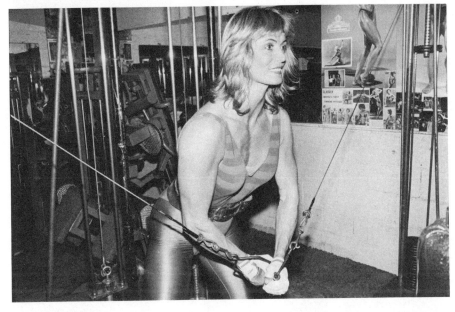

Finish.

Cable crossovers stress the whole pectoral muscle complex, particularly the inner and lower sections. Bodybuilders do cable crossovers to etch striations across their pectorals.

CABLE CROSSOVERS
Exercise Emphasis

Grasp the handles attached to a pair of high pulleys, your arms extended upward at approximately a 45-degree angle from the floor on each side. Set your feet at about shoulder width, rotate your palms downward for the entire set, and bend slightly forward at the waist.

Starting Position

Slowly move your hands downward in semicircular arcs until they touch each other about six inches in front of your body. Hold this position momentarily while tensing your pectorals as hard as possible. Allow your hands to return to the starting point, and repeat the movement for the desired number of repetitions.

Movement Performance

Many bodybuilders prefer to do this exercise while kneeling on the floor, a variation that isolates the legs from the movement. You can also do crossovers with one arm at a time.

Exercise Variations

BACK EXERCISES

DUMBBELL SHRUGS
Exercise Emphasis
All forms of shrugs directly stress the trapezius muscles. Secondary stress is on the forearm and upper chest muscles.

Starting Position
Grasp two moderately heavy dumbbells, and stand erect with your arms hanging down at your sides. Sag your shoulders downward and slightly forward.

Movement Performance
Shrug your shoulders upward and to the rear as high as possible. Lower the dumbbells back to the starting point, and repeat the movement for a suitable number of repetitions.

Exercise Variations
You can do rotating dumbbell shrugs. In this movement you shrug your shoulders in circles—upward, backward, downward, and forward. You can also perform rotating shrugs in the opposite direction.

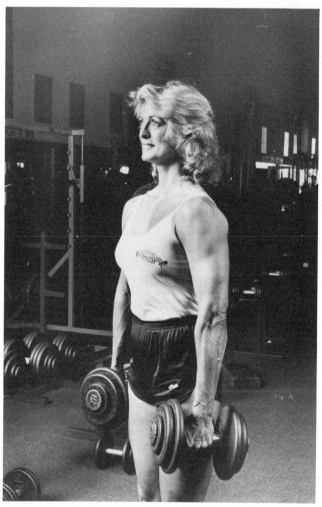

Start.

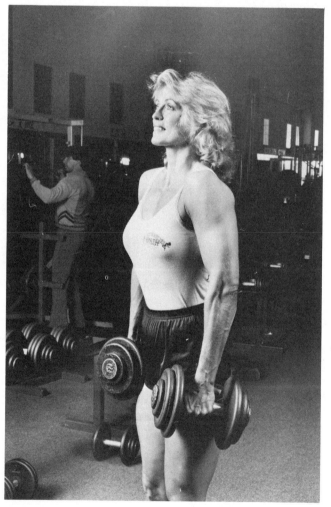

Finish.

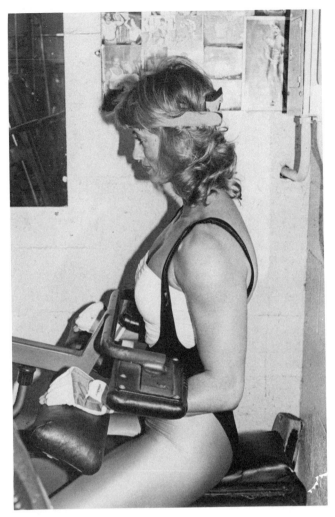

Nautilus start.

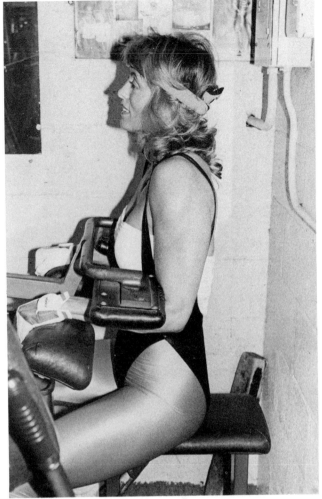

Nautilus finish.

Machine shrugs directly stress the trapezius and forearm muscles. Secondary resistance is placed on the upper chest muscles.

Stand between the handles of the bench press station of the gym unit. You can either face toward the weight stack or away from it. Grasp the handles of the pressing lever arm, and stand erect with your arms held straight throughout the movement. Sag your shoulders downward as far as possible.

Sit on the seat of the shrugging machine, and run your forearms between the two pads on each side of the machine. Sag your shoulders downward as far as you can.

Forcefully shrug your shoulders as high as possible. Lower the machine back to the starting point, and repeat the movement for the required number of repetitions.

Most women need to stand on a 4 × 4-inch block of wood when doing shrugs on a Universal machine. Standing on the block ensures that you still have resistance on your working muscles at the bottom point of the movement.

MACHINE SHRUGS
Exercise Emphasis

Universal Gyms
Starting Position

Nautilus Starting
Position

Movement Performance

Exercise Variations

165

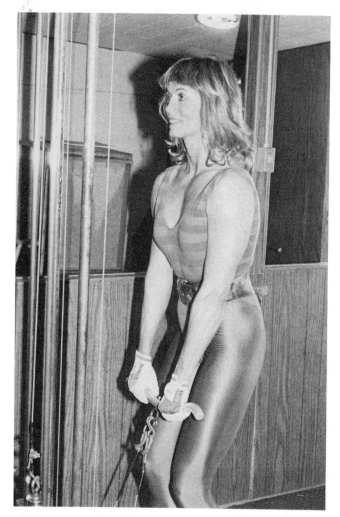

Start.

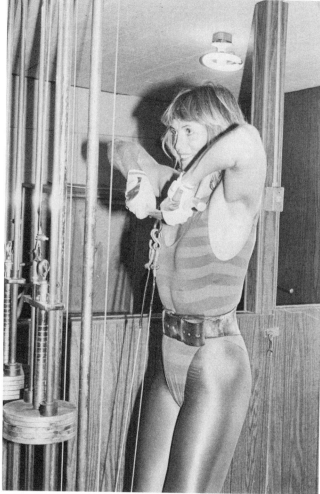

Finish.

PULLEY UPRIGHT ROWS
Exercise Emphasis

All forms of upright rowing place primary stress on the deltoids and trapezius. Secondary emphasis is on the forearm and biceps muscles.

Starting Position

Attach a short bar handle to the cable running through a floor pulley, and take a narrow overgrip on the handle. Stand erect with your toes about six inches back from the pulley and fully straighten your arms.

Movement Performance

Keeping the bar no more than an inch or two from your torso on its upward journey, slowly pull the barbell upward until it touches the underside of your chin. As you pull the barbell upward, your elbows should be well above the level of your hands. Lower the barbell back to the starting point and repeat the movement.

Exercise Variations

You can vary your grip width on the handle when doing cable upright rows.

Stiff-legged deadlifts intensely stress the erector spinae and hamstring muscles and place secondary stress on the forearm and upper back muscles.

STIFF-LEGGED DEADLIFTS
Exercise Emphasis

Grasp a moderately weighted barbell with a shoulder-width overgrip. Stand erect with it. Lock your arms and legs straight throughout the movement.

Starting Position

Slowly bend forward at the waist to lower the barbell to as low a position as comfortably possible.

Movement Performance

To achieve a longer range of motion, you should stand on a flat exercise bench or thick block of wood. When standing on a bench or block, you can lower the barbell farther without the plates touching the floor and thus terminating the downward movement of the barbell.

Exercise Variations

Start, done standing on a bench.

Finish.

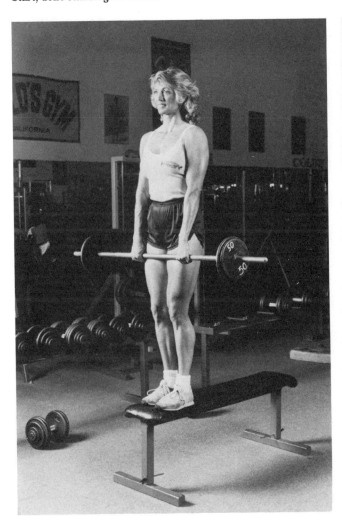
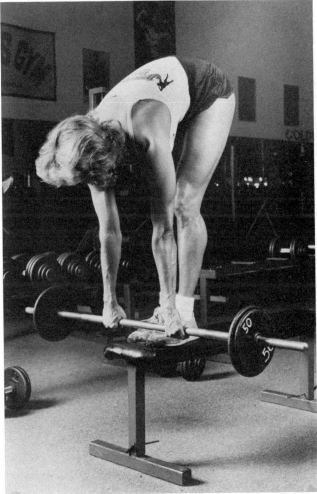

| "GOOD MORNINGS" Exercise Emphasis | This movement intensely stresses the erector spinae and hamstring muscles. |

"GOOD MORNINGS"
Exercise Emphasis   This movement intensely stresses the erector spinae and hamstring muscles.

Starting Position   Place a light barbell across your shoulders and behind your neck, balancing it in position by grasping the bar near the plates on each side. Place your feet about shoulder-width apart, and keep your legs locked throughout the sets.

Movement Performance   Slowly bend forward at the waist until your torso is slightly below a position parallel with the floor. Return to the starting point, and repeat the movement for the required number of repetitions.

Exercise Variations   Many women prefer to do "good mornings" with legs slightly bent and/or to a position well below an imaginary line parallel to the floor.

Patsy Chapman demonstrates the starting position.   ...and the finish.

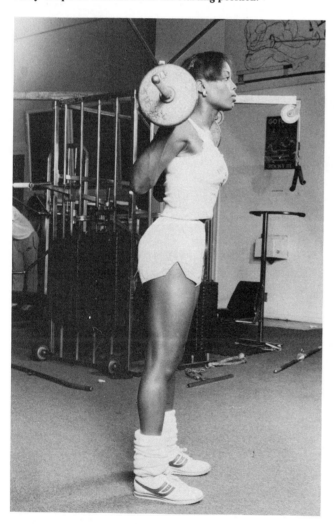

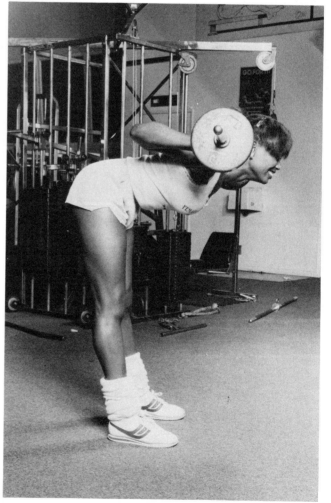

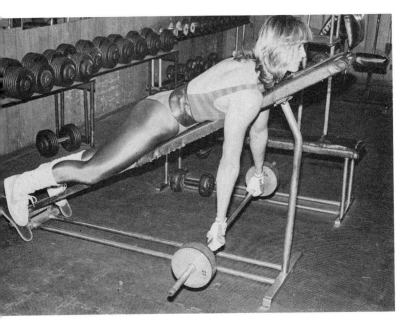

Start, using bench set at an incline.

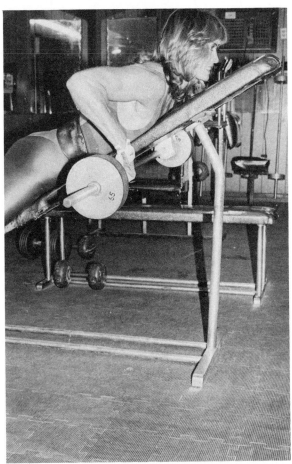

Finish.

Bench rows strongly stress the latissimus dorsi, the back portion of the deltoids, the biceps, the brachialis, and the forearm muscles. Since it is performed with the torso supported, it can be done to add to upper back thickness even when the lower back is sore.

Adjust a flat exercise bench to a level that allows you to straighten your arms at the bottom of the movement without the barbell touching the floor. Lie facedown on the bench, and have two training partners hand you the barbell so you can take an overgrip slightly wider than shoulder width on the bar. Straighten your arms fully.

Making sure that your upper arms travel to the rear, slowly pull the barbell directly upward until it touches the underside of the bench. Return the weight to the starting position, and repeat the movement for the required number of repetitions.

You can elevate either end of the bench a few inches higher than the other end when you do bench rows. Each of these bench angles will stress your back muscles somewhat differently.

BENCH ROWS
Exercise Emphasis

Starting Position

Movement Performance

Exercise Variations

169

SHOULDER EXERCISES

FRONT RAISES
Exercise Emphasis

Front raises place primary emphasis on the frontal deltoids and secondary emphasis on the middle section of the delts.

Starting Position

Place your feet at shoulder width, grasp two light dumbbells, and stand erect with your arms hanging down at your sides. Straighten your arms and keep them straight throughout the movement. Turn your hands so your palms are facing the rear.

Movement Performance

Slowly raise your right hand in a semicircular arc up the midline of your body until it is slightly above shoulder level. Begin lowering the dumbbell in your right hand, and commence raising the weight in your left hand. Continue alternately raising and lowering the dumbbells until you have done the required number of repetitions with each arm.

Exercise Variations

This movement can be done with a single dumbbell held in both hands. You should wrap a towel around the dumbbell and hold the handle so it is perpendicular to the floor in the top position of the movement. You can also do front raises holding a barbell in both hands. Most bodybuilders take a shoulder-width grip on a barbell, but you can experiment with narrower and wider grips.

Left arm at full extension.

Right arm at full extension.

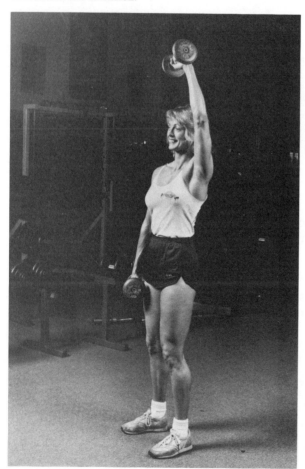

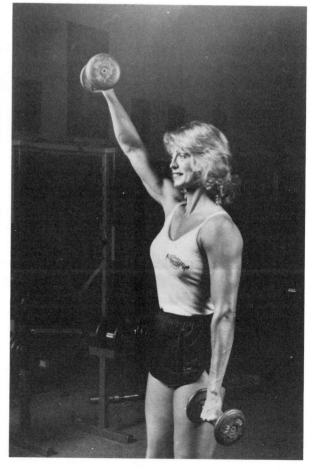

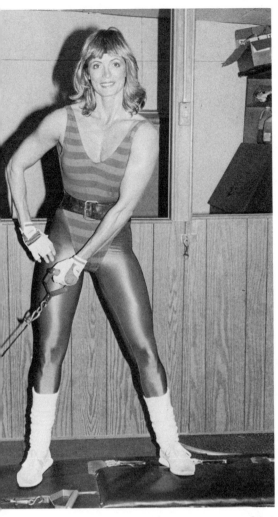

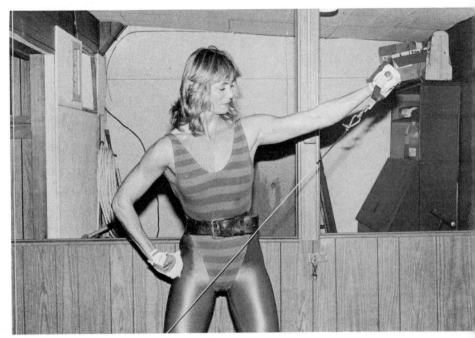

Finish.

Start.

You can isolate stress primarily on the medial deltoid heads using cable side laterals. Minor secondary stress is placed on the front part of the deltoids.

CABLE SIDE LATERALS
Exercise Emphasis

Grasp a loop handle attached to a cable running through a floor pulley with your left hand. Stand erect with your right side facing the pulley, the cable running diagonally across your body, and your right foot about three feet from the pulley. With your palm facing the pulley, move your right hand to a position about six inches directly in front of your right hip. Bend your left arm slightly and keep it bent throughout the movement.

Starting Position

Slowly move your left hand in a semicircle from the starting point to shoulder height out to the left. Lower your hand back along the same arc to the starting point, and repeat the movement for an appropriate number of repetitions. Repeat with your right arm.

Movement Performance

You can do this exercise with the cable running diagonally across your body behind your back, or with your right hand when your right side is toward the pulley.

Exercise Variations

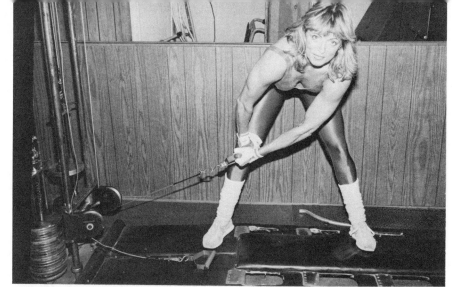

Using one arm (start).

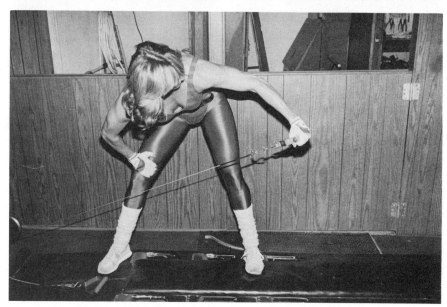

Finish.

CABLE BENT LATERALS
Exercise Emphasis

Cable bent laterals strongly stress the posterior deltoid heads and place secondary stress on the medial delts and trapezius muscles.

Starting Position

Stand between two floor pulleys with your feet set about shoulder-width apart. Reach toward the right pulley with your left hand, and grasp a loop handle attached to the cable. Move to the left and grasp the loop handle of that pulley in your right hand. Bend over until your torso is parallel to the floor, and cross your arms beneath your torso. As you do the movement, the cables will cross each other directly beneath your torso if you are in the correct starting position.

Movement Performance

Slowly move your hands in semicircular arcs directly out to the sides until your hands are a bit above shoulder level. Lower your hands back along the same arcs to the starting point and repeat the movement.

Exercise Variations

You can do this movement with one arm at a time, the cable passing beneath your body as you do the exercise.

Prone incline laterals strongly stress the medial and posterior deltoid heads. Secondary stress is placed on the anterior deltoids and trapezius muscles.

Grasp two light dumbbells and lie facedown on a 45-degree incline bench. Hang your arms directly downward and bend them slightly. Touch the dumbbells together directly beneath your shoulders, your palms facing each other.

Starting Position

Raise the dumbbells directly out to the sides and upward until they are slightly above shoulder level. Lower the dumbbells back along the same arcs to the starting point, and repeat the movement for the required number of repetitions.

Movement Performance

To place additional stress on the anterior deltoids, you can raise the dumbbells directly forward rather than out to the sides.

Exercise Variations

Start.

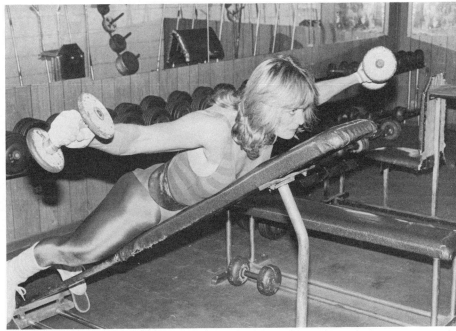

Finish.

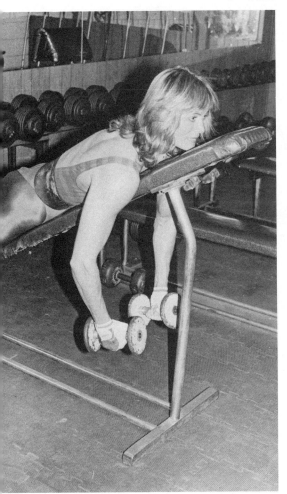

173

ARM EXERCISES

PREACHER CURLS
Exercise Emphasis

Preacher curls primarily stress the biceps muscles, particularly the lower third of the muscle group. Secondary stress is placed on the powerful flexor muscles of the forearms.

Starting Position

Take a palms-up grip on a barbell, with your hands set two or three inches wider than your shoulders on each side. Run your upper arms down the angled surface of a preacher bench, holding them parallel to each other. Fully straighten your arms.

Movement Performance

Slowly bend your arms as fully as possible to move the barbell in a semicircular arc from the starting point until it is under your chin. Lower the barbell back along the same arc to the starting point, and repeat the movement for the required number of repetitions.

Exercise Variations

You can do this movement with two dumbbells held in your hands, or with one arm at a time.

Arms extended.

Arms flexed.

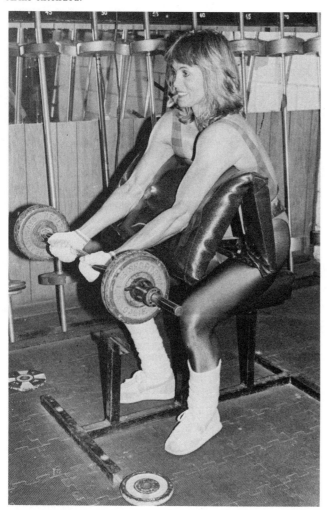

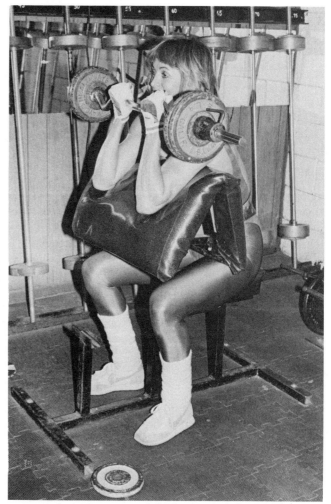

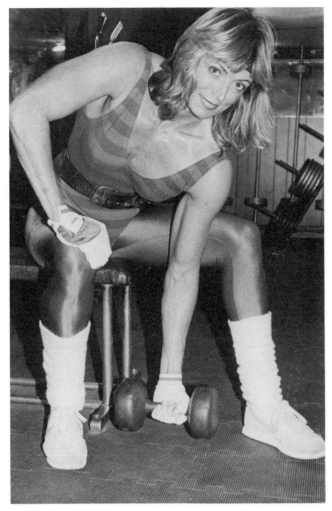

Start.

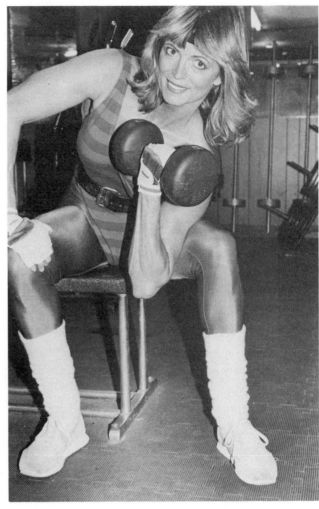

Finish.

This movement places primary stress on the biceps muscles and secondary emphasis on the flexor muscles of the forearms. Bodybuilders do concentration curls to add to the peak on their biceps.

Sit at the end of a flat exercise bench and place your feet about shoulder width on the floor. Grasp a light dumbbell in your left hand, straighten your arm, and place the back of your exercise arm against the inside of your left thigh near your knee. Place your right hand on your right knee, or brace in against your left thigh behind your left arm. Turn your left hand until your palm is toward your right leg.

Starting Position

Slowly bend your left arm as fully as possible to curl the dumbbell up to your shoulder. Slowly lower the weight back to the starting point and repeat the movement. Be sure to do the same number of sets and repetitions for each arm.

Movement Performance

You can do this movement bending over at the waist so that your torso is parallel to the floor, your working arm is hanging straight down from your shoulder, and your free hand is placed on a bench to brace your body in position during the movement.

Exercise Variations

175

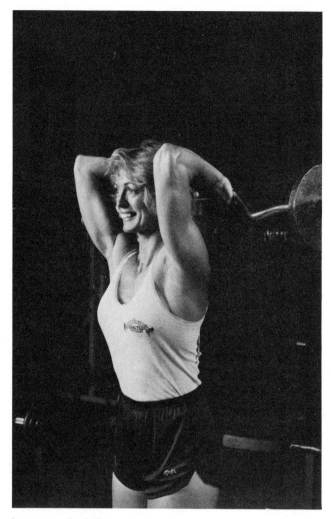

Start, using barbell.

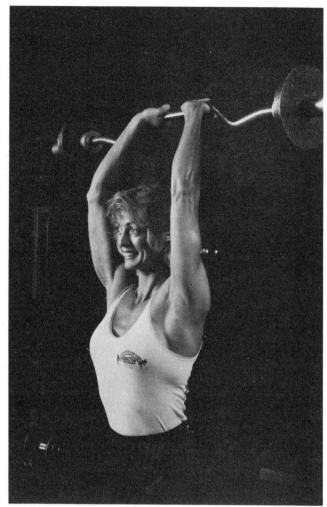

Finish.

STANDING TRICEPS EXTENSIONS
Exercise Emphasis

All forms of triceps extensions strongly stress the triceps muscles and place secondary emphasis on the muscles of the forearms.

Starting Position

Take a narrow overgrip on a barbell (there should be about six inches of space between your hands). Pull and push the barbell to straight arm's length above your head.

Movement Performance

Keeping your upper arms motionless, slowly bend your arms and lower the barbell in a semicircular arc from the starting position downward until it touches your neck. Slowly return it along the same arc to the starting point, and repeat the movement for an appropriate number of repetitions.

Exercise Variations

You can perform triceps extensions with a single dumbbell held in both hands, or with one arm at a time while holding a dumbbell. When holding a single dumbbell in both hands, your palms should be flat against the under side of the top plates of the dumbbell, and the handle of the dumbbell should hang perpendicular to the floor during the movement.

176

All forms of triceps extensions strongly stress the triceps muscles and place secondary stress on the muscles of the forearms.

Take a narrow overgrip on a barbell (there should be about six inches of space between your hands). Lie back on an incline or decline bench, and extend your arms directly upward from your shoulders.

Starting Position

Keeping your upper arms motionless, slowly bend your arms and lower the barbell in a semicircular arc downward until it touches your forehead. Slowly return it along the same arc to the starting point, and repeat the movement for the required number of repetitions.

Movement Performance

You can vary the width of your grip and/or use a reversed grip on all triceps extensions.

Exercise Variations

Incline extension, start.

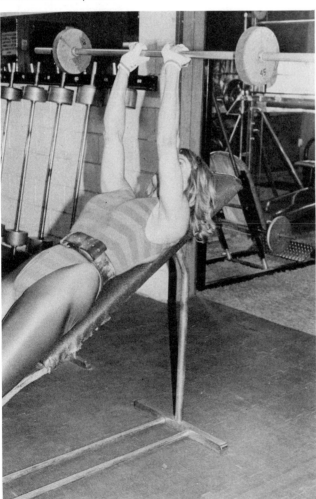

Finish.

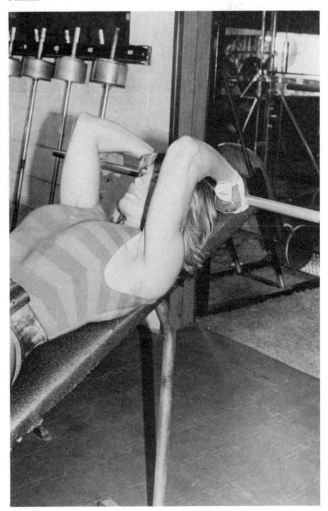

DUMBBELL
KICKBACKS This is an excellent movement for stressing the triceps in relative isolation from the rest
Exercise Emphasis of the body.

Starting Position Grasp a light dumbbell in your left hand, bend over until your torso is parallel to the floor, and brace your body in position by resting your right hand on a flat exercise bench. Press your left upper arm against the side of your torso in a position parallel to the floor, and bend your arm at a 90-degree angle.

Movement Performance Keeping your upper arm pressed against your torso, slowly straighten your arm as fully as possible. Lower the dumbbell back to the starting point and repeat the movement.

Exercise Variations You can do this movement with both hands holding dumbbells.

Start, bracing free hand on knee.

Finish.

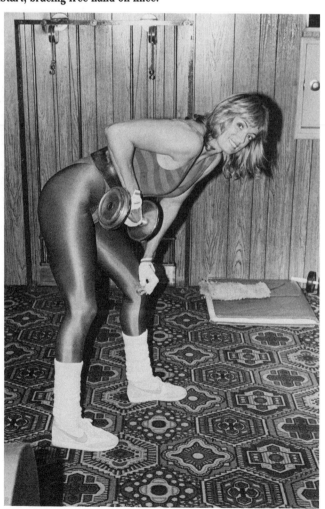

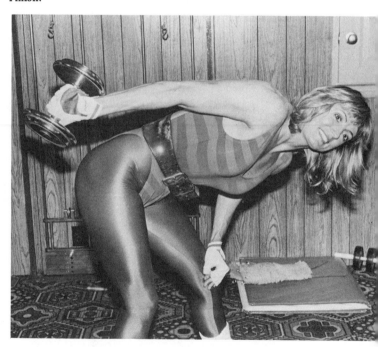

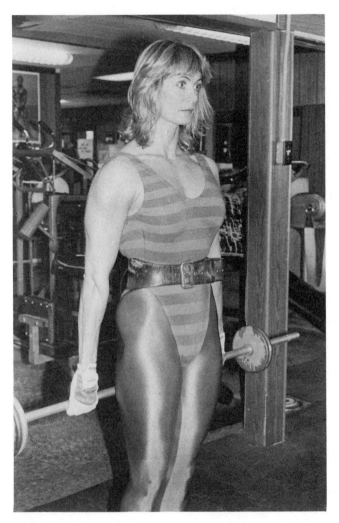

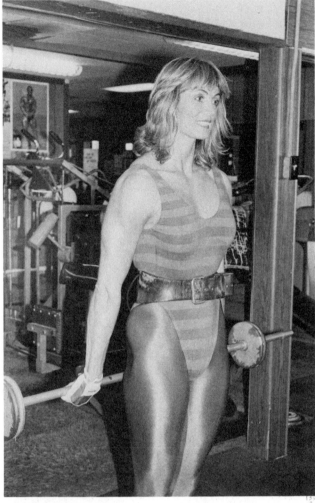

Start.   Finish.

Standing wrist curls strongly stress the powerful flexor muscles on the insides of the forearms.

STANDING WRIST CURLS
Exercise Emphasis

Place a barbell across a high exercise bench. Back up to it and take a shoulder-width grip on the barbell, with your palms facing the rear. Stand erect, with your arms straight and the barbell resting against your upper thighs behind your back.

Starting Position

Slowly flex your wrist to curl the barbell backward and upward in a small semicircular arc to as high a position as possible. Slowly lower the barbell back to the starting point, and repeat the movement for an appropriate number of reps.

Movement Performance

You can do this movement while holding two dumbbells in your hands with your palms facing each other.

Exercise Variations

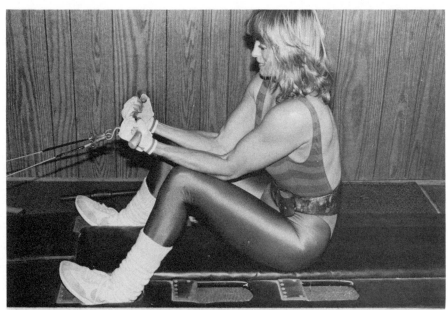

Palms-up position.

Palms-down position.

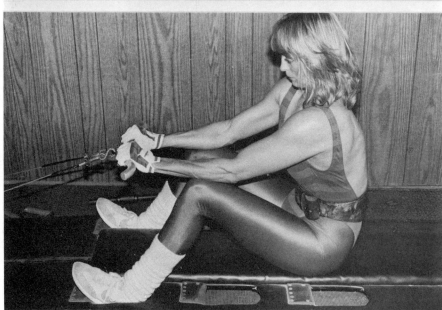

PULLEY WRIST CURLS
Exercise Emphasis

Performed with your palms up, pulley wrist curls stress the flexor muscles of the forearms. Done with your palms down, the movement stresses the extensor muscles of the forearms.

Starting Position

This movement can be done identically on either a free floor pulley or the low pulley of a Universal Gyms machine. A similar movement can also be done by attaching a short handle to the end of the lever arm of a Nautilus multipurpose machine. Sit at the end of a flat exercise bench, place your feet at shoulder width on the floor, take an undergrip on a handle attached to the pulley cable, and run your forearms down your thighs so your fists hang off the edge of your knees. Sag your fists downward as far as possible.

Movement Performance

Flex your wrists to curl the handle slowly in a small semicircular arc to as high a position as you can. Lower the handle back to the starting point and repeat the movement.

Exercise Variations

You can also do this movement with your palms facing the floor. Regardless of the variation, you can vary the width of your grip on the handle for slightly different stresses on the forearm muscles.

180

CALF EXERCISES

This movement strongly stresses the gastrocnemius muscles of the calves.

NAUTILUS MULTI MACHINE
Exercise Emphasis

Fit the hip belt around your waist just above your hips with the metal ring attached to it hanging in front of your body. Attach the ring to the hook at the end of the machine's lever arm. Step up on one of the steps of the machine, placing only the toes and balls of your feet on the step. Your feet should be about shoulder width apart, and your toes should be pointed directly forward. Sag your heels as far below the level of your toes as you can.

Starting Position

Slowly rise up as high as possible on your toes. Return to the starting position, and repeat the movement for an appropriate number of repetitions.

Movement Performance

As with all calf exercises, you should also do sets with your toes angled outward at about 45 degrees on each side, as well as angled inward. You can also vary the width of your foot placement.

Exercise Variations

Start.

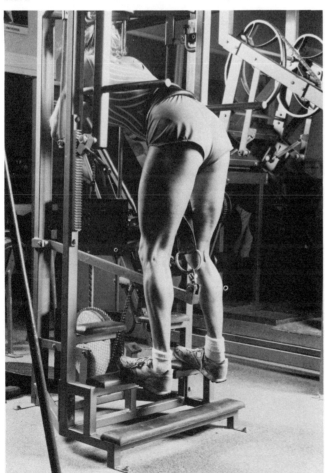

Finish.

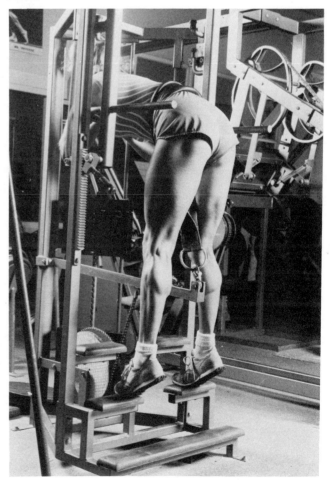

MIDSECTION EXERCISES

HANGING FROG KICKS
Exercise Emphasis   Frog kicks stress the frontal abdominal muscles, particularly the lower section of the rectus adbominis muscle complex.

Starting Position   Jump up and grasp a chinning bar, with a grip slightly wider than your shoulders. Hang your body straight below the bar.

Movement Performance   Slowly bend your legs and pull your knees up to touch the lower edge of your rib cage. Return your body to the starting point, and repeat the movement for the required number of repetitions.

Exercise Variations   You can involve your intercostals by twisting your torso to each side on alternate repetitions. If you find it difficult to keep your torso from swinging as you perform the exercise, you can have a training partner grasp the sides of your waist to hold your torso motionless.

Start, using a parallel bar alternative.

Finish.

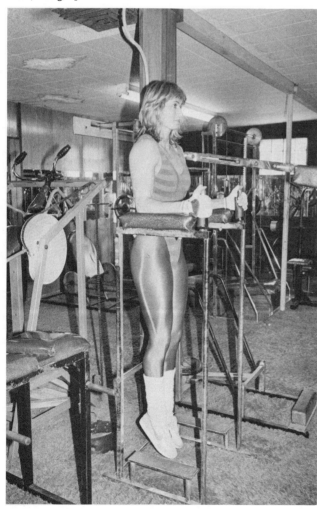

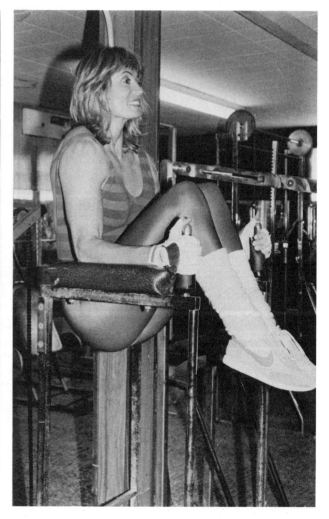

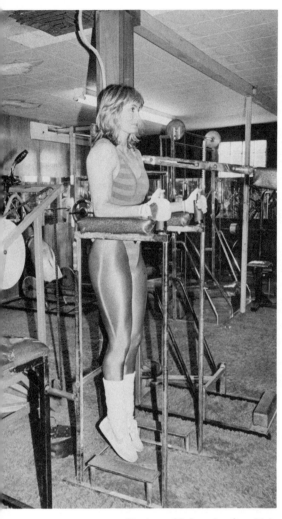

Start as with hanging frog kick.

Finish.

Hanging leg raises intensely stress the frontal abdominal muscles, particularly the lower section of the rectus abdominis muscle complex.

HANGING LEG RAISES
Exercise Emphasis

Jump up and grasp a chinning bar, with a grip slightly wider than your shoulders. Hang your body straight below the bar, and bend your legs slightly.

Starting Position

Slowly raise your feet in a semicircular arc from the starting point to a position slightly above the level of your hips. Lower your feet back to the starting point, and repeat the movement for the desired number of repetitions.

Movement Performance

If your abdominal muscles are very strong, you can raise your feet up to the level of the bar. Should you find it difficult to keep your torso from swinging as you perform the movement, you can have a training partner grasp the sides of your waist to hold your torso motionless.

Exercise Variations

183

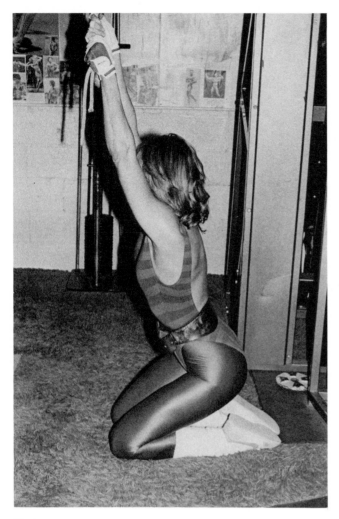

Start.

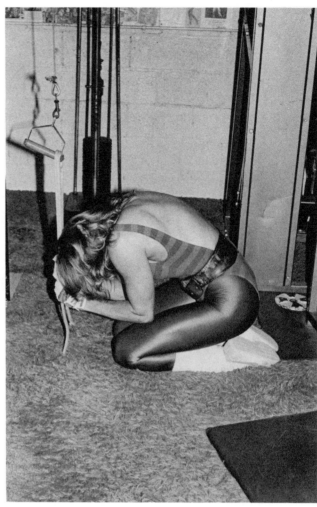

Finish.

ROPE CRUNCHES *Exercise Emphasis*	Rope crunches directly stress the rectus abdominis muscle group, particularly the upper section.
Starting Position	Attach a rope handle to the cable running through a high pulley. Grasp the ends of the rope, and kneel on the floor about two feet back from the pulley. Straighten your arms and extend them toward the pulley. Incline your torso toward the pulley.
Movement Performance	Bend forward until your forehead touches the floor, at the same time bending your arms and pulling the rope handle down to touch the floor an inch or two in front of your head. Forcefully exhale while doing the exercise. Return to the starting point, and repeat the movement for the desired number of repetitions.
Exercise Variations	You can bring your intercostal and serratus muscles into action by twisting your torso a bit to each side on alternate repetitions. You can also do this movement using a short bar handle.

184

LEVEL THREE WORKOUT

You should push every post-warm-up set to failure when doing the exercises in the following routine. Also gradually increase the number of sets on which you use forced reps.

MONDAY/THURSDAY

Exercise	Sets	Reps
1. Hanging leg raises	2–3	20–30
2. Roman chair sit-ups	2–3	20–30
3. Seated twists	2–3	50
4. Machine incline presses	2	6–10
5. Decline flyes	2	8–12
6. Nautilus flyes	1	8–12
7. Seated presses behind the neck	2	6–10
8. Cable bent laterals	2	8–12
9. Cable side laterals	1	8–12
10. Dumbbell shrugs	2	10–15
11. Pull-downs behind the neck	2	8–12
12. Seated pulley rowing	2	8–12
13. Front pull-downs	1	8–12
14. "Good mornings"	2	10–12
15. Standing barbell wrist curls	2	10–15
16. Pulley reverse wrist curls	2	10–15
17. Nautilus multi calf raises	2	10–15
18. Seated calf raises	1–2	10–15

TUESDAY/FRIDAY

Exercise	Sets	Reps
1. Bench leg raises	2–3	20–30
2. Rope crunches	2–3	15–20
3. Seated twisting	2–3	50
4. Squats	2	10–15
5. Leg extensions	2	10–15
6. Leg curls	2	10–15
7. Partial squats	1	10–15
8. Barbell preacher curls	2	8–12
9. Dumbbell concentration curls	1	8–12
10. Barbell reverse curls	1	8–12
11. Incline triceps extensions	2	8–12
12. Dumbbell kickbacks	2	8–12
13. Pulley wrist curls	2	10–15
14. Barbell reverse wrist curls	2	10–15
15. Standing calf raises	2	10–15
16. Calf presses	1–2	10–15

MY PERSONAL WORKOUT ROUTINE | 9

The preceding chapters present workout strategies for the beginner and the intermediate and advanced bodybuilder. While I have personally followed the programs presented there and received substantial benefit from them, I have found that what works best for me is a three-days-per-week total-body workout routine. And that is the program I will describe in this chapter.

This is a very complicated workout pattern based on the latest evidence on how muscles most readily hypertrophy. However, as the evidence is not all conclusive, an element of personal experimentation remains.

The program was largely developed for me by my coach, Jerry Doyle, of Phoenix, Arizona. This gentleman, now in his mid-sixties, is a former world champion high diver. For many years he was a professional acrobat, and he's worked in the health and fitness industry for most of his life. It's through observation of athletes he's trained or seen train under the tutelage of others that he developed my training program. Compared to the more traditional methods outlined in the preceding chapters, his program for me is quite radical.

At first I did not want to adopt this training program—I was afraid it was too different and that I would not succeed with it. I was wrong. I grew from being an "also ran" competitive bodybuilder to winning a national championship within twelve months' time. And now that I am a resident in orthopedic surgery and soon to become a full-time orthopedic surgeon busily involved in my own practice, the three-day-per-week training regimen is most convenient. As of this writing, I am on call the other two weekdays and every other weekend and could not possibly handle a training program that required my presence in the gym four to five days per week every week. (I do make the time sacrifice when getting ready for a contest. Then I work out five or even six days a week, usually after 10:00 P.M. or before 6:00 A.M.)

I work out on Tuesdays, Thursdays, and Saturdays. Each workout begins with the same series of warm-up exercises. I perform a few minutes of light jogging, rebounding on a trampoline or stationary cycling. I then move quickly to a bench and perform 200 seated twisting exercises while grasping a long broom handle. I begin gradually. Usually the first few reps are accompanied by the readjustment of the vertebrae in my lower back; **187**

I can hear them snap into realignment. It feels good to get the kinks out of my back. The intensity of the twists becomes progressively greater, and by the time I have done 50 to 60 of them, I am able to twist quite vigorously from side to side without fear of injury.

After completing the twists, I move to the hanging leg-raise machine and do six sets of twenty hanging leg raises. I rest only enough between sets to catch my breath and to let the burning sensation in the abs subside so that I can complete the twenty reps in the next set.

I then do seated calf raises or standing calf raises—whichever I do not perform in the beginning of my workout, I perform later at the end. I usually begin with the seated calf raises, because in the beginning an exercise I can perform sitting down has slightly more appeal. I perform a warm-up set with a very light weight, progress to a slightly heavier weight for another twenty reps, then perform five or six sets with very heavy weight, doing as many reps as I can—usually from fifteen to seventeen. I keep my rest periods short—about fifteen seconds—to let the burning sensation in my calves subside enough so I can begin the next set.

Then I call my coach, Jerry, over to the chest machine because I am ready to begin my workout. Mental attitude is very important here. I am usually grouchy at this point. I am often tired and impatient. I don't want to waste time in the gym, as I still have reading and things to do for the next day once I get home. It bothers me when others are clowning around in the gym. But instead of complaining or fussing, I channel all my energy into working as hard and heavy as I possibly can. So I begin very seriously. I have to. The workout will be three hours long, and there is no leeway for slack energy levels.

TUESDAY'S WORKOUT

THE CHEST AREA   I begin my workout proper with *flyes performed on the Nautilus machine.* (Descriptions of most of the exercises I'll mention here are given in the preceding chapters.) I do a warm-up set of four to five reps with light resistance (40 to 50 pounds), do one rep at an intermediate weight (80 pounds), and a next at 100 pounds. Then I move to a heavy weight of 120 pounds for one rep and up again to 130 pounds for the next rep or two. Then I go to 140 pounds, after which I try to break my own weight record—two reps unaided at 140 pounds. I try 145 or 150 until I get failure. Following that I drop down to a weight at which I can do eight reps before failure (110 to 120 pounds).

Sometimes minimal assistance may be needed with one arm or the other at completion, but I refuse help from my coach until I absolutely cannot move the weight. I want every ounce of benefit from the workout, which means doing as much as possible on my own. Finally I'll let Jerry help me push out a last three or four reps. It's true that fatigue of itself does not build muscles, but I believe that extra demand placed on them in this way to keep working does stimulate some growth. The muscle adapts according to the demand placed on it, particularly if the stress is repeated regularly.

After a fifteen-second rest pause, I progress into what we call "singletons," single reps using the same weight as in the previous set. I do from ten to fifteen of them. Then, with Jerry's help, I force an extra five reps, so I can barely move when I've finished. Everything hurts so much; the pump I feel is terrific.

After a recovery period of no more than two minutes, I progress to a set of negatives. I pull the weight up. Jerry stands on the foot support of the machine, grasps hold of the

bars just above where my hands are placed, and pushes back while I resist with all my might. This puts tremendous strain on the pectoral muscles at their insection on the sternum (breastbone) and really helps add to the definition that I have in this area. It also increases muscle thickness here.

I do the next phase of my chest workout on *the bench press portion of the pec-deck machine.* I follow the same progression, working up to a maximum weight one rep at a time, then going to a set of ten to twelve reps, followed by singletons and then by negatives.

The negatives are done on a Nautilus machine specially built for negative chest work. (I'm very fortunate that Jerry Doyle's gym has this piece of equipment. Most Nautilus facilities don't.) With this exercise, the number of negative reps runs from fifteen to twenty. I set the machine at 150 to 180 pounds. This is the equivalent of 300 to 360 pounds of free weight. If I were doing this exercise as a regular bench press, it would be like lowering a bar with upwards of 300 pounds of weight on it. (I couldn't possibly lift that much, but could manage lowering it. I could do the best second half of a bench press in the world, if that counted for anything.)

The third phase of my chest workout uses another unusual piece of apparatus, *the dynamic tension machine, or infometric bench.* It has a bench that can be raised to three different heights in order to give you inclines, declines, and flat benches. The machine has two handles that are grasped in a bench press kind of position, and you provide your own resistance. I provide my own resistance with one hand while pushing as hard as possi-

Working the chest muscles with the dynamic tension machine.

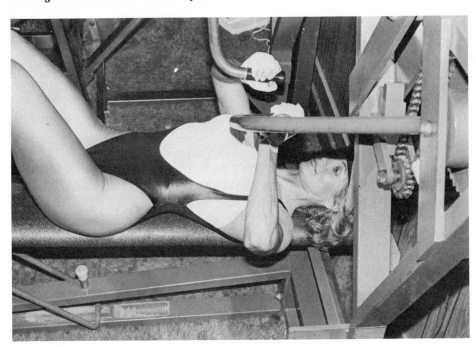

ble with the other through a movement that calls for complete elbow extension and horizontal shoulder flexion, as in a typical bench press action. When the pushing arm has reached full extension, it provides the resistance for the other, which now pushes the same way in its turn.

This series of alternating movements against resistance is great for isolating the muscles of the chest, one pectoral at a time. It is also excellent for working the middle and outer heads of the triceps.

I perform fifteen reps with each arm in each of the three positions—incline, decline, and flat. The entire sequence takes about ten minutes, and it is the physiological equivalent of doing over fifty sets of chest work.

What really makes this series potent are the singletons I perform right after the first heavy set. The muscles are allowed to rest only enough after each to bring them to the level of a last repetition before failure on a very heavy set. That is often the rep in which the most effort is expended. This makes the singletons a series of maximum contractions with very heavy load, which is the type of stimulus most likely to lead to muscle hypertrophy.

THE BACK   I move to the *Nautilus pullover machine* for my first back exercise. Again, I begin with a light warm-up set of approximately five to six reps with resistance at 50 pounds. Then I progress through intermediate weights into a series of single maximum-effort exertions, followed by ten to twelve reps using the heaviest weight I can work with to complete the set. Jerry helps me force out the last few reps. (The weight at this point is somewhere between 130 and 150 pounds.)

Following the progression previously described, I next do a set of singletons and then a series of negatives—from twelve to fifteen reps.

I move from the pullover machine to the *pull-down machine,* positioning myself so that I am pulling the weight from about one foot in front of me rather than directly over my head. I follow the same progression of maximum-effort reps, a series of heavy singletons, and a set of negatives.

From the pull-down machine I go to the *Nautilus machine for developing the rear deltoids and the trapezius* and, with Jerry's help as needed, follow the same progression.

After that I do *Nautilus lat presses.* These are performed while sitting on the Nautilus lat press machine. The arms are extended above the head to rest against the rollers. Then, with the weight set at from 70 to 80 pounds, I pump out two sets of fifteen reps.

From there I progress to the pulleys and do *seated cable pulley rows* using 110 to 130 pounds of weight. I do three sets of from eight to twelve repetitions each. I make sure the pulley level is adjusted to encourage low back involvement, which stimulates strength development in the lower back and erector spinae muscles.

Once I've done these, I've completed by back exercises. I congratulate myself for having made it past the row of machines I call "Death Row," because the chest and back workouts are the most exhausting part of my routine.

THE SHOULDERS   I do the first shoulder exercise on the *Nautilus double shoulder machine.* I begin with *lateral raises,* following the format of progression to maximum effect with heavy sets (weight resistance is from 100 to 110 pounds), followed by singletons and negatives.

Then I do *military presses on the Nautilus deltoid machine.* The weight here is from 80 to 90 pounds. The number of repetitions on the heavy set is from ten to fifteen. I often need more help on this machine than on any of the others.

I do the negatives on a Nautilus machine specially developed for negative military presses. The negative machine (and this is true of the one designed for chest negatives, too) is designed so that you push the weight out with your feet. The weight should be heavy enough so that it overpowers you and you're doing the best you can just to resist it coming down. You may even have to keep your feet on the foot pedal so as not to be so totally overpowered that the weight comes crashing down. The exertion here really counts for muscle growth. I use approximately 120 to 150 pounds resistance, which is the equivalent of 240 to 300 pounds of weight pressing down on my shoulders. I do twelve to twenty reps ordinarily, more when I am in preparation for competition.

THE ARMS

For biceps development, I use the *Nautilus biceps curl machine,* which works both arms at the same time. There are no handles to hang on to, just pads against which to rest your wrists. That prevents you from using your forearms to move the weight. Only your biceps should be working to flex your arm; the forearm muscles that insert above the elbow should not be brought into play. The elbows should be high on the corresponding pad, and you should make sure that they go through the full range of motion from complete extension to complete flexion.

I vary the usual progression here by doing a heavy set right at the beginning, with the weight at about 10 pounds under the maximum I will use on my heavy set after doing single reps to failure. This is to "pre-exhaust" the muscle, priming it for maximum contraction with the singletons. Then I follow with the heavy set of eight to twelve reps, which is in turn followed by ten to fifteen singletons. The rest interval between singletons is very brief—five to fifteen seconds—just enough to let me contract the muscle and pull the weight up again. The last singletons are forced out with assistance from Jerry, although only enough to allow completion of the movement, as maximal muscle contraction must be obtained.

Depending on my particular needs and the time, I may do *another set of arm exercises* on a somewhat older Nautilus machine that I think works better than some of the newer ones. It is heavier and has foot pedals on it that allow me to do negatives on my own if Jerry is not around. All I have to do is load the machine up with more weight than I can pull toward me, use my legs to help push the weight up, and then take my feet off the pedals and resist the downward motion as best I can using my triceps. I follow the same sequence as with the biceps movements, doing a pre-exhaustion set before working to a maximum weight effort. Then again the set of reps at a slightly lower-than-max weight, followed by the series of singletons.

THE LEGS

I start my leg workout with *leg extensions.* First I do a warm-up set with 80 pounds and then work up to 200 pounds, with one or two reps at each intermediate weight. That's followed by a set of one-two-three attempts at a maximal one-rep effort. (I've done up to 270 pounds on the leg extension machine.) Then I do one set of fifteen reps using 240 to 250 pounds, followed by twenty singletons and twenty negatives.

On the negatives, I use about 200 pounds. I perform the leg extension and then hold the legs extended while Jerry pushes down to force me to flex at the knees. I resist all the way, even after he's overcome the full leg extension, so that the weight lowers slowly.

I find that I have to do more reps with the leg exercises, because the leg muscles seem to require higher reps for growth than do the upper body muscles. Also, as it takes a long time for an extensor leg muscle to reach maximal contraction, the speed at which the exercises is completed is slower than for the upper body. Because the weight used is so

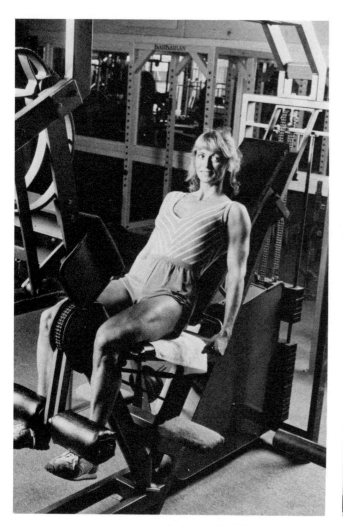
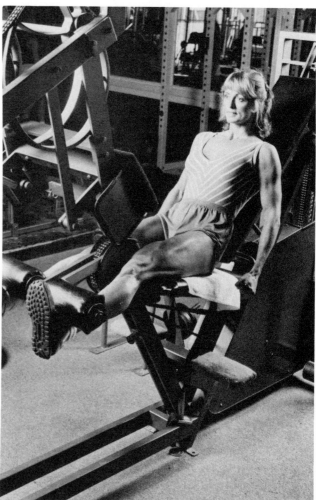

Leg extensions done on the Nautilus leg extension machine.

heavy, I usually put pads between my shins and the roller of the leg machine in order to ease the pressure on my shins.

After the leg extensions, I do *hamstring curls* on the leg machine—a warm-up set with 60 pounds, intermediates of 80 and 90 pounds, a maximum-effort single, and then a workout weight of from 100 to 110 pounds for a heavy set of from fifteen to twenty reps. Those are followed by fifteen or so singletons and fifteen to twenty negatives. Jerry supplies the resistance for the negatives by pulling on the roller apparatus at the end of the machine while I resist as hard as I can with sustained knee flexion.

Following the hamstring curls, I do *leg presses on the Nautilus leg press machine.* I place a four-inch thick cushion behind my back. This helps bring my hips into a position where my gluteals are emphasized more than my quadriceps. I get as close to the machine as possible and perform a warm-up set with 110 pounds. Then I perform a set of fifteen to twenty reps using 170 to 190 pounds, followed by twenty singletons done quickly. I do not do negatives in this exercise.

My fourth leg exercise is one on the *Nautilus hip/back machine.* By this time I don't need a warm-up—it would probably make me too tired to finish the exercise. I go immediately to as heavy a weight as I can use and work each leg individually. The weight is set at 100 pounds, and I do three sets of ten reps for each leg.

I've found working on this machine particularly benefits my upper hamstring development. When I was preparing for the recent American championships, both Jerry and I were surprised at the muscle that showed through when I began to drop weight in eliminating body fat. In women, fat tends to concentrate around the upper thigh area, and I am no exception when it comes to that. But after I'd dropped 10 to 15 pounds, this new area of development was remarkably apparent, and I attribute it to use of this machine.

The last leg exercise is a calf workout, usually *standing calf raises* or *donkey-style calf raises done on the Nautilus multipurpose machine.* I set the weight at anywhere from 150 to 200 pounds for five or six sets of from fifteen to twenty reps each. While I do standing calf raises on a fairly regular basis, I find that they put a lot of pressure through my shoulders into my lower back, and I often avoid this exercise for that reason.

My warm-up routine actually incorporates a first exercise for the abs, hanging leg raises. **THE ABDOMEN**

Now near the end of my workout, I use the *Nautilus abdominal machine* to perform six sets of twenty reps each with the weight resistance set at 110 pounds. I could use more weight, but I find that it bothers my back to do so, primarily because of the strain occasioned by initially pulling the weight up or letting it down. Jerry will help with the initial movement for that very reason.

Because my abs are very thick and I do not want them to overwhelm the symmetry of my waistline, I limit my abdominal workout to the warm-up hanging leg raises and work on the Nautilus ab machine. I haven't been doing sit-ups for more than two years. I've found that sit-ups build a wide, flat waist. As a result of my current routine, my abs have been thicker than ever, my intercostal development has been better than ever, and my waist remains small. There's actually been a noticeable decrease in my waistline from just over twenty-five inches to around twenty-four inches now. The twists I do during my warm-up play an important role in this, too.

I do two or three sets of negatives on the Nautilus abdominal machine with Jerry's assistance. I pull up 80 pounds and then try as hard as I can to hold that up as Jerry overpowers me by pushing down to force me to extend at the waist. We stop the motion before I get to complete extension so that we don't risk injury to the lower back. We do ten reps for each set.

When you try this series of movements for the abs, you will find that your abs get very sore the first time or two, no matter what kind of exercise you've been doing previously. So be very careful, especially on the negatives.

I do *curls* and *wrist extensions* on the Nautilus multipurpose machine, with three sets of **THE FOREARMS** each, performing ten to fifteen reps per set. And when I've completed those, I've finished my regular Tuesday workout.

THURSDAY'S WORKOUT

On Thursday I work out primarily with free weights. The entire workout features supersets aimed at working a particular body part and its opposing "antagonist." (Supersets, you will recall, are two exercise sets performed without a rest break in between to stress opposing muscle groups.) I start with the same warm-ups as on Tuesday.

I use the Nautilus multipurpose machine for the first sequence in the workout itself, *pull-ups.* I do ten to twelve reps in free sets, supersets with *dips,* and then another fifteen pull-up reps.

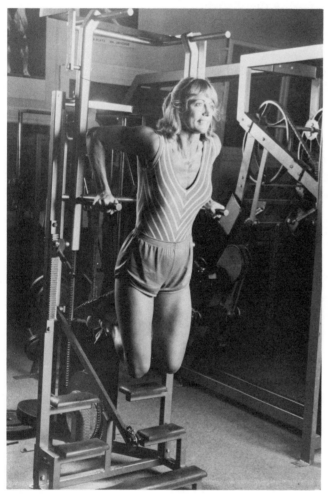

Doing dips.

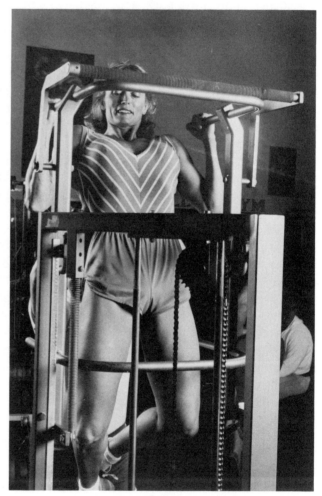

. . . and pull-ups (chins) in a superset.

After this, I do *seated military presses* with 40-pound dumbbells. This again is a superset. I perform eight to ten reps and then immediately go to a set of *behind the neck pull-downs,* performing twelve to fifteen reps with 130 pounds of weight.

The third exercise combination consists of *incline dumbbell bench presses* supersetted with a *lat pull-down* variation. The presses are done with 45- to 50-pound dumbbells for eight to twelve reps. Then the lat pull-down is performed leaning back with the legs hooked under at the T-bar that is fastened to the floor. The pull-down is to the level of the chest. The weight used is 140 pounds for fifteen reps.

194

If I use a barbell, the weight is from 130 to 140 pounds. It's ten reps for either. The lat pull-downs are done with a palms-up grip, holding the hands together. The weight used is from 130 to 140 pounds. This pull-down variation emphasizes the biceps as well as the lats.

The fifth superset duo features *standing arm curls* using either heavy dumbbells in alternation or an easy curl bar, followed immediately by *close-grip bench presses* performed with the easy curl bar. The curls are done with as heavy a weight as possible for ten to twelve reps (counting each paired alternate movement as a single rep). The bench press, done for long triceps extensions, is also done with as heavy a weight as possible for ten to twelve reps. I do three supersets.

Then I go to *long cable bicep curls,* supersetted with *standing cable triceps extensions.* Here, too, I use as heavy a weight as possible for completing from fifteen to twenty reps, and I concentrate on achieving a cramping motion in either biceps or triceps with each repetition, depending on the exercise.

The seventh exercise set is a free set of Smith squats, without a complementary superset of another movement. I use the Smith machine when performing very heavy squats because doing them with a barbell puts an uncomfortable, possibly dangerous strain on my lower back. I use upwards of 180 pounds on the Smith machine, usually somewhere around 220 pounds, and do from twelve to fifteen reps. I place my hands on my knees at the beginning and end of the movement to protect my knees as I go all the way down and to assist in pushing myself up. Taking this precaution, I don't have to put on knee wraps.

. After the Smith squats, I go back to supersetting, using the inner/outer thigh machine produced by Nautilus. I do twenty reps with 80 pounds for both abduction and adduction, performing from three to five sets, depending on whether I'm in precompetition training or not.

The last regular part of my Thursday routine is a series of either seated or standing calf raises—whichever I didn't perform in my warm-up—following the Tuesday format, and then abdominal work on the Nautilus ab machine—six sets of twenty reps at 110 pounds. I don't do negatives on these abdominals on Thursdays.

Sometimes I do additional forearm work, but I often don't. Most of the heavy weight workout done on Thursdays involves a tremendous amount of forearm work anyway.

SATURDAY'S WORKOUT

On Saturdays I perform the same exercises as on Tuesday, making this again a workout heavily oriented to use of the Nautilus machines. However, I don't follow the same pattern of progression through each movement.

The object on Saturday is to put maximum stress on all the muscle fibers, including those known as the slow-twitch red fibers. Conventional workouts stress primarily the two other types of muscle fiber—the fast-twitch red and fast-twitch white fibers. (The "twitch" reference indicates speed of reaction to a contraction stimulus. It takes a more sustained stimulus to force the slow-twitch fibers into maximum contraction.) My Saturday workout, which is the most exhaustive of the three regular weekly routines, aims at promoting maximum growth throughout the entirety of each muscle. The workout itself takes about two and a half to three hours. The idea is to work all the muscle groups to a point of total burnout.

The exercises are done in the same order as on Tuesday, but a reverse kind of princi-   **195** ple is followed. Instead of warming up to a maximum effort in each movement via a set of intermediate-weight reps, I go to the heaviest possible weight immediately after the usual warm-up set. For example, on the double pec machine, I do flyes with the maximum weight of around 130 pounds for five to eight reps and then do a downward progression—a next set of eight to ten reps with 10 pounds less weight, quickly followed by a set of ten reps with the weight again 10 pounds lighter, and so on until I've completed five sets, doing ten reps per set on the last three or four sets. Then a final set is done with twenty reps, even if it takes assistance from Jerry to force out the final four or five.

In some cases we'll follow this exhausting round with a set of negatives, but most of the time we do not. We're more likely to do negatives for the chest and back than the arm, shoulder, or abs. If you're trying to build up mass in the chest and back, I recommend that on Saturday you do the same negatives as prescribed for the Tuesday workout. I also do negatives on the leg extensions and leg curls frequently, in line with my observation that the leg muscles seem to need more work to stimulate hypertrophy.

In the Saturday workout I move quickly from machine to machine with very little rest between exercises. This is because I want to get an aerobic effect by keeping the heart rate up and to subject slow-twitch red muscle fibers to maximum stress.

I make it a point to do a full-body routine on Saturday. It is the most exhausting of the routines, and finishing it on Saturday allows me all of Sunday and Monday to recover for Tuesday's workout. If for some reason I'm forced to break the routine short—to do one part of it on Saturday and the other on Sunday—I'm never quite as strong on Tuesday.

PRECONTEST ADJUSTMENTS IN ROUTINE

When I'm preparing for a contest, I have to follow a schedule of training five or six days a week to gain that competitive edge. I start six weeks ahead of the event by incorporating thirty to ninety minutes of bike riding into my daily activity routine. And I go to the gym on my usual off days (Monday, Wednesday, Friday) to work on my abdominals and calves. The calf work is important, because I have a tendency to slight my calves if I'm pushed for time in a workout. I have to make up the difference before the contest is on.

As I get down to the four-week mark, I begin to work my legs every day, particularly with the extension and curl machines and the hip/back extension machine. The last-named has proven invaluable to me in cutting up my thighs. I also try to do the Nautilus inner/outer thigh machine at least four times a week to rid myself of any fatty deposits in the upper inner thigh area.

This kind of schedule is very tough, because I also have patients to attend to at the hospital. However, I have a key to the gym, so have no excuse of a lack of facilities when I finally do have time. Only complete physical exhaustion will keep me from going to the gym. But I only compete three or four times a year, because the schedule is so demandingly difficult. I can't afford more than three or four months of competition prep time. I also group my contests within that period so I don't have to go through this distracting intensive routine throughout the year.

Even during my precompetition training period, I do not run more than twice a week. I was at one time a track athlete and love to run, but I've found that running drastically depletes my upper body. My arms, shoulders, back, and chest will thin out, and months of hard training will be lost if I insist on running more than three days a week or more than three miles at a shot.

Bike riding is fine, but that has to be kept to a reasonable minimum, too. The high reps in pedaling can help to thin the legs out more than is desirable at a point where you want mass.

The key to the success of my program is the watchful eye of my coach, Jerry Doyle. He observes not only my muscularity, but my symmetry, too. We avoid exercises that thicken the waist—particularly lots of heavy squats, deadlifts, and powerlifting. A lot of women respond well to these exercises, and if you are one of them, then let the exercises work for you. But I find that they give me a more masculine line than I want. My goal is to have an optimally muscled feminine physique. Whatever prizes they may hand out in a contest, the highest reward for me is always achieving the strong, feminine line I envision for myself. I have built what I wanted to build.

Every woman who undertakes a bodybuilding regimen should keep that in mind— she is striving for a goal that is very personal, very individual. If maximum muscularity is your goal, then you have every right to go after that. Do not feel that you have to adopt some other person's or group's goal to justify your training. I have a great deal of respect for women bodybuilders with goals of maximum muscular development. They train very hard, and they have an audience in the bodybuilding public. I do not share their goal; I prefer a different look. That is a matter of personal choice, growing out of my own esthetic. You may prefer my look; you may prefer the heavily muscled look. Whichever you prefer, let what you envision for yourself above all be your own look.

APPENDIX

Drugs and Bodybuilding

The idea in bodybuilding is improve your general state of health and to develop the musculo-skeletal system to optimum potential. To me that implies a sport emphasizing what is natural to the body and rejecting any artificial means of stimulating growth or regulating body function. Your body is a finely tuned instrument capable of maintaining itself in balance and of simultaneously achieving tremendous physical potential through athletic effort. Via controlled diet and a regimen of exercises pushing your body to fulfillment of genetic potential, you can accomplish wonders.

But increasingly in this day and age, one finds people relying on the shortcut of drug use to achieve athletic goals. While the short-term effects are often impressive, over the long range this kind of shortcutting can cost bitterly. There are substantial health risks involved. And even when it seems a matter of only "slight risk" of impaired function or development, that price does not look to be worth it. Where is the advantage in sacrificing even a little of your health over the long term?

It isn't only a matter of actual physical damage, on whatever scale. Drug use has an inevitable mental effect as well. An athlete finds she cannot train, let alone compete, without relying on drugs. She develops a dependence on them; she does not actually face up to the challenge of putting her own resources fully to the test. She fears inadequacy on that score. And meanwhile the delicate balance of chemistry in the body is disturbed, making it all the more likely that she compromises whatever chance she has of ever proving her *own* potential to herself.

When it comes to drug use in bodybuilding, the specific questions revolve primarily around the use of anabolic steroids to stimulate muscle hypertrophy, the use of diuretics to eliminate unwanted water from the system, and the use of diet pills for weight control purposes. In each case an athlete using them makes the drug part of the overall athletic program. The use of recreational drugs can have serious health consequences, too, but their use grows out of a pursuit of different goals. Resorting to and dependence on recreational drugs is a subject best viewed in the context of a general psychological orientation to life and its demands and opportunities. A discussion of that is beyond the scope of this book—except for the warning that drug use is not compatible with a health-oriented bodybuilding lifestyle. What makes it necessary to discuss the drugs noted above at greater length is the fact of a dangerous paradox in the training philosophy of some who state a commitment to the bodybuilding lifestyle. They claim to focus attention on the body's optimum development while undermining that in pursuit of a short-term advantage.

Let's look at the three drug use areas for a clear understanding of the implications in each.

ANABOLIC STEROIDS

A lot of people think that all the leading figures in competitive bodybuilding use anabolic steroids. And why not? Haven't the men been using them for years and getting fantastic results?

To begin with, let me assure you that the top women in bodybuilding do not rely on anabolic steroids for their development. If you look at how they've developed themselves over the past four or five years, you will see that it's been a matter of consistent hard training over an extended period of time. Those are not sudden gains made as a result of drug use. It is not the established champions who are into drugs. It is invariably the new woman impatient to make her mark in the sport who asks me, what about anabolic steroids?

Anabolic steroids are synthetic male hormones. They have two effects, not just one. In addition to the anabolic effect—building muscle size and strength—they have what is known as an androgenic effect. They influence the development of the secondary sex characteristics associated with males—a deeper voice, increased facial hair, increased muscularity, susceptibility to male pattern baldness, increased hemoglobin levels in the blood, heavier bones, a more masculine body line, and more widespread distribution of body hair. While the synthetic hormones are designed to heighten the anabolic effects and minimize the androgenic effects, there is no synthetic male hormone that is wholly free of the androgenic side effects.

These drugs come in two forms—one to be taken orally, one to be injected intramuscularly. (There are, however, many different formulations available in either form.) Regardless of how they enter the body, anabolic steroids act on all tissues of the body. The musculo-skeletal tissues are particularly sensitive to their effects, but so are the hormone-sensitive receptors on the ovaries and in the pituitary and hypothalamus glands. And other organs show significant sensitivity, too.

Research shows that anabolic steroids have a "positive" effect on the body's nitrogen balance. The increase in available nitrogen appears to contribute to the development of muscle mass and strength. But this effect has not clearly been established, and other studies suggest that the drugs have primarily a psychological effect as far as muscle growth is concerned. It has been shown that anabolic steroid ingestion by animals increases levels of aggression, and it may be that in humans a similar effect leads to more aggressive workouts. Since the drug, to be effective, must be combined with heavy training and a high protein intake, it may well be the latter more than the former that really stimulate the extra growth.

A regimen including use of anabolic steroids increases the number of red blood cells, with a consequent greater amount of hemoglobin to carry oxygen to the working muscle. This sounds like a great advantage, but in fact if too many red blood cells are produced, a condition known as polycythemia results. The blood cells start to clog up the capillaries supplying nutrients to various of the vital organs, for example, the spleen and the heart.

200   I know of an athlete who was taking anabolic steroids over a period of several years who ran into this problem. He became quite ill. He was able to regain his health through good medical care, but he suffered some permanent damage to various organs in his body.

Other side effects include an increase in water and salt retention, which would be very dangerous for anyone with high blood pressure or high levels of saturated fatty acids and/or cholesterol in the blood. These side effects would be most threatening to anyone with a family history of coronary heart disease.

Very little of the research done on the effects of anabolic steroids has involved women. Studies on dosage and effect have almost all been conducted with male subjects. However, certain body mechanisms for maintaining a chemical balance are common to both men and women, so the results shown in males almost certainly will be evident in women.

It appears that a dosage of upward of 50 mg. per day has to be used to get the full anabolic effect (assuming there is that effect as a result of using the drug, whether directly or indirectly). The body has its own sense of the proper hormone level, so it gradually adapts to a given dosage. In order to maintain the "advantage" of an increased hormone level, one actually has to step up dosages regularly or the body adjusts to where there is essentially no added response. You might start off with 2 mg. per day, but you have to build that intake up to 10 mg. and then to 20 mg. and so on in order to continue the accelerated-development effect.

It's also because of your body's compensating reaction in this fashion that you cannot come off anabolic steroids cold turkey. The body's natural hormone production system has been slowed or shut down, particularly the adrenal glands and the ovaries, which produce the bulk of the sex-related hormones. When the synthetic hormone is withdrawn abruptly, the body is left in a state where it has no hormone for available use. The glands are not in a state to immediately produce what is needed. You will experience a withdrawal effect, particularly an adrenal crisis, which can be life-threatening. Anyone who has been taking synthetic hormones is advised to taper off slowly to allow the glands to be stimulated into restoring function gradually rather than be shocked by a sudden demand they cannot meet. (This advice is offered for those who are stupid enough to experiment with these drugs despite cautions to the contrary.)

There's an important additional consideration for women—the possible effect on the reproductive system and the implications of use in conjunction with the possibility of having children. There may be an interruption in the menstrual cycle while taking anabolic steroids. Perhaps more significantly, there may be an effect on children not yet born.

Every egg in the ovary that you will have for ovulation and for the formation of future children is present at your birth. That means every egg is there while you are taking anabolic steroids and vulnerable to any effect from them. No one knows how the normal development of a child may be affected as a result, but there is concern about possible dangers. It seems clear that if a woman is pregnant and takes anabolic steroids at that time, there is extreme danger of hyper-masculinization of the fetus. That can be tragic, especially when it's a female child.

There's some question about whether anabolic steroids are any better or worse if taken orally as opposed to being injected. The oral drugs are absorbed directly into the blood's mainstream from the intestine. This takes them directly to the liver, where they are largely metabolized (burned off) or inactivated before they can get to the muscle where the desired benefit is to occur. The injectibles go directly into the whole network of blood vessels/arteries rather than up a quick one-way street and so will reach muscle tissue without first being processed by the liver. On the other hand, the injectibles diffuse into the system more slowly, and they are more easily detected in drug tests.

DIURETICS

There are bodybuilders who use diuretics, particularly in connection with competition preparation, to tap off "excess" water so they get a very cut-up look to their physique. There are some who go so far as to combine the use of dangerous diuretics with other dehydrating procedures such as exercising in rubber suits, sitting in saunas, or simply not replenishing the normal loss of body fluids.

Diuretics use can be very dangerous. The decreased blood flow could result in renal eschemia, death of parts of the kidney that didn't get enough oxygen because of reduced flow. These drugs can also deplete the electrolytes in the body, particularly potassium, and this may lead to irregular heart rhythms, which are dangerous in turn because of the greatly increased risk of heart attack. I know of several instances of fatalities as a result of the use of diuretics such as Lasix in a non-medically prescribed fashion.

A mild herbal diuretic or one that spares potassium may help someone who is retaining water in a premenstrual period or who has an unusually high level of female hormones, which can cause water retention. But even these should not be used on a continual basis by an otherwise healthy individual.

The best way to get rid of water in the system is to drink eight to ten glasses of water per day. This stimulates regularity on the part of the kidneys. Accustomed to a steady intake of water, the kidneys will establish a balance level for fluids in the body that does not entail holding on to a reserve. When you deplete yourself of fluids, the kidneys take a compensatory precaution. Water that is subsequently taken into the system will be retained to provide something of a reservoir against the next shortage. As little as possible will be flushed through via the urine; you may get very concentrated urine. In fact, testing the specific gravity of urine before a competition could be one way of monitoring diuretics use. The higher the specific gravity, the more likely it is that the individual has been dehydrating too severely or using diuretics to achieve a dehydrated state.

In my opinion, the competitive look that one gets from excessive dehydration is not attractive. The person looks cut up even when she is not flexed, and the impression is of a stringy kind of muscularity. I prefer a smoother look when one is relaxed. Then when you flex your muscles, they jump out readily through a skin that is lean from dieting, not dried out from abuse of diuretics.

I firmly believe that one reason Rachel McLish as been so successful as a bodybuilder is her reliance on maintaining a natural balance in her body's working. She trains and diets in a most healthful manner. She does not use drugs in an effort to win a competitive advantage. Her look onstage is distinctly a cut above that of others. She appears smooth when standing relaxed, but when she flexes, all the muscle groups are there and nicely displayed. This is most attractive and has provided her an edge over others who may look more symmetrical or more muscular but don't radiate the same kind of healthful appeal. Hers is a true beauty, and I think we will find that it is the look that wins most consistently in our sport as judges become more keenly observant of the effects provided by fundamentally unhealthy practices such as reliance on diuretics.

DIET PILLS

Diet pills, whether they be amphetamines or non-amphetamines available by prescription, are used by some to help them get through periods of controlled food intake. They have the seemingly marvelous effect of depressing the appetite and lifting one's spirits while on a diet, particularly a precompetition diet that is low in carbohydrates. (As you will recall from my comments in Chapter 2 of this book, I strongly advise against a low-carbohydrate diet, even though it tempts many a bodybuilder.)

The problem with using diet pills is not only that you develop a psychological dependence on the drug for keeping control of your diet, but also that you will gain weight more easily afterwards. Once you stop taking the diet pill, your appetite becomes ravenous. I have seen many women who have taken diet pills and obtained marvelously cut-up physiques for competition show up with thirty to forty pounds of excess fat three months later. I've tried diet pills myself—a non-amphetamine variety—and discovered that my weight came back in no time after a contest and that I wound up fatter than I was before.

The reason for the rebound effect with use of diet pills is, once again, the body's own sense of balance. Basically, a diet pill is an "upper." Now, the central nervous system knows what the activation level of the body should be and works to maintain that level through whatever you may do to change it—in this case, by adding stimulants. When you take diet pills on a regular basis for any length of time, the central nervous system makes a compensating adaptation. It reduces its own output of natural stimulants to metabolism. To get the heightened effect on a continuing basis, you actually have to keep increasing your intake of the drug.

When you stop taking diet pills after a period of reliance on them, the stimulating effect provided is withdrawn. Meanwhile, your body's own natural level of activation has been depressed; you're operating with a reduced metabolic rate all of a sudden, because the body's own natural stimulants are no longer being produced at the level normal for you. This temporarily lowered metabolism facilitates rapid weight gain. So all that you worked for is quickly lost.

You may feel that it was worth it for a chance to win, but I think it makes bodybuilding a progressively more difficult sport if you wind up always having to fight huge swings in weight. You have to have some fat on you in order to become more muscular. You can't be in lean, cut-up shape between competitions and still increase your muscularity as effectively as if you have a normal, healthy fat reserve, say 18 to 20 percent of body weight. With that normal fat reserve, you can build muscle more readily while on a controlled diet that drops the body fat down to 8 to 10 percent for contest performance, which may require only four to five weeks. That reduced fat level can fairly easily be maintained for another four to five weeks. You can compete in two or three contests within a one-month period, take a rest, and then get yourself ready again for another two or three contests. This is what I did in 1982. I went on a diet for four to five weeks, using my normal reserves to build muscle mass and strength, and competed in good shape in a couple of contests within the same month. I didn't have to rely on diet pills to get me to a goal weight or to reduce the proportion of fat in my body. Sensible reliance on my body's innate capabilities and on my own sense of discipline and self-control carried me through. And I didn't have to deal with the unpleasant side effects that come with reliance on a drug.

To me, that's what bodybuilding is all about. It's not just a question of fairness, although that is an appropriate consideration when it comes to deciding on the admissibility of drug use. More fundamentally, I believe that drug use is simply contrary to any lifestyle that emphasizes achievement of healthful physical potential. It is self-defeating in the long run to use any substance that throws off the body's own balance mechanisms in an effort to get the best out of one's body. The shortcuts to seeming advantage provided by drug use are all too often the fast road to impaired function and reduced potential.

BIBLIOGRAPHY

BOOKS

Anatomy

Gray, Henry. *Anatomy, Descriptive and Surgical.* London: Crown Publishers, 1968.

Bodybuilding

Combes, Laura, with Reynolds, Bill. *Winning Women's Bodybuilding.* Chicago: Contemporary Books, Inc., 1983

Kennedy, Robert. *Natural Body Building for Everyone.* New York: Sterling Publishing Co., Inc. 1980.

Murray, Jim. *Inside Bodybuilding.* Chicago: Contemporary Books, Inc., 1978.

Pearl, Bill. *Keys to the Inner Universe.* Pasadena, CA: Physical Fitness Architects, 1979.

Schwarzenegger, Arnold, with Hall, Douglas Kent. *Arnold's Bodyshaping for Women.* New York: Simon and Schuster, 1979.

Sprague, Ken, and Reynolds, Bill. *The Gold's Gym Book of Bodybuilding.* Chicago: Contemporary Books, Inc., 1983.

Weider, Joe, with Reynolds, Bill. *The Weider System of Training.* Chicago: Contemporary Books, Inc., 1983.

Weider, Joe (editor). *Women's Weight Training and Bodybuilding Tips and Rountines.* Chicago: Contemporary Books, Inc., 1982.

Weider, Joe, and Weider, Betty. *The Weider Book of Bodybuilding Tips and Routines,* Chicago: Contemporary Books, Inc., 1982.

Flexibility

Anderson, Bob. *Stretching.* Fullerton, CA: Anderson-World, Inc., 1975.

Injury Treatment and Rehabilitation

Mirkin, Gabe, and Hoffman, Marshall. *Sports Medicine Book.* Boston: Little, Brown & Co., 1978.

Kinesiology

Wells, Katharine E., and Luttgens, Kathryn. *Kinesiology: Scientific Basis of Human Motion.* Philadelphia: W. B. Saunders Co., 1976.

Nutrition

Darden, Ellington. *The Nautilus Nutrition Book.* Chicago: Contemporary Books, Inc., 1981.

Neve, Vickie. *Pat Neve's Bodybuilding Diet Book.* Phoenix, AZ: Phoenix Books, 1980.

Nutrition Almanac. New York: McGraw-Hill Book Co., 1977.

Physiology

Astrand, Per-Olof, and Rohdahl, Kaare. *Text Book of Work Physiology.* New York: McGraw-Hill Book Co., 1977.

Weight Training

Barrilleaux, Doris, and Murray, Jim. *Inside Weight Training for Women.* Chicago: Contemporary Books, Inc., 1978.

Darden, Ellington. *The Nautilus Book* (Revised). Chicago: Contemporary Books, Inc., 1982.

Dobbins, Bill, and Sprague, Ken. *The Gold's Gym Weight Training Book.* Los Angeles; J. P. Tarcher, Inc., 1977.

Ferrigno, Carla. *For Women Only: Carla Ferrigno's Total Shape-Up Program.* Chicago: Contemporary Books, Inc., 1982.

Murray, Jim. *Contemporary Weight Training.* Chicago: Contemporary Books, Inc., 1978.

Murray, Jim. *Winning Weight Training.* Chicago: Contemporary Books, Inc., 1982.

Reynolds, Bill. *Complete Weight Training Book.* Mountain View, CA: Anderson-World, Inc., 1976.

Reynolds, Bill. *Weight Training for Beginners.* Chicago: Contemporary Books, Inc., 1982.

Sing, Vanessa. *Lift for Life!* New York: Bolder Books, 1977.

Sprague, Ken. *The Gold's Gym Book of Strength Training.* Los Angeles: J. P. Tarcher, Inc., 1979.

Zane, Frank, and Zane, Christine. *The Zane Way to a Beautiful Body.* New York: Simon and Schuster, 1979.

MAGAZINES

Bodybuilder. Charlton Publications, Charlton Building, Derby, CT 06418.

Body & Power. Family Publications, Box 1984, Reseda, CA 91335.

Flex. 21100 Erwin St., Woodland Hills, CA 91367.

Iron Man. Box 10, Alliance, NE 69301.

Muscle Digest. 10317 E. Whittier Blvd., Whittier, CA 90606.

Muscle & Fitness. 21100 Erwin Street, Woodland Hills, CA 91367.

MuscleMag International. Unit Two, 270 Rutherford Rd. S., Brampton, Ontario L6W 3K7, Canada.

Muscle Training Illustrated. 1665 Utica Ave., Brooklyn, NY 11234.

Muscle Up. Charlton Publications, Charlton Building, Derby, CT 06418.

Muscle World. Charlton Publications, Charlton Building, Derby, CT 06418.

Muscular Development. Box 1707, York, PA 17405.

Strength & Health. Box 1707, York, PA 17405.

FEDERATION ADDRESSES

American Federation of Women Bodybuilders, Doris Barrilleaux, Box 937, Riverview, FL 33569.

International Federation of Bodybuilders, 2875 Bates Rd., Montreal, P.Q. H3S 1B7, Canada.

KEEP FIT WITH WARNER BOOKS

IMPORTANT BOOKS FOR YOUR BODY
FROM WARNER BOOKS

M.J. SAFFON'S YOUTHLIFT   (L97-816, $4.95, U.S.A.)
                                               (L37-274, $5.95, Canada)

How to firm your neck, chin, and shoulders with minutes-a-day exercises. The no-surgery natural way to looking younger longer. Prevent the signs of age... banish them if they've begun...erase them and look young again.

M.J. SAFFON'S BODY LIFT   (L37-363, $5.95, U.S.A.)
                                               (L37-921, $7.25, Canada)

The no-exercise, no-diet way to reshape your body and regain your skin's youthful beauty. Reshape your body contours—eliminate love handles, bra bulges, thigh sags! Banish skin discoloration—lighten weathered red skin, darkened body area! Smooth skin texture—correct gooseflesh, aging elbow roughness, swelling, puffiness!

THE 5-MINUTE-A-DAY NATURAL WAY TO YOUNG EYES
M.J. Saffon   (L38-007, $3.50, U.S.A.)
                                               (L38-009, $4.25, Canada)

A quick, simple, safe program of exercises and eye care for beautiful, youthful eyes. M.J. Saffon, beauty consultant to the world's most famous women, presents the best, safest, least expensive way to give your eyes the look of youth without surgery!

THE 15-MINUTE-A-DAY NATURAL FACE LIFT   (L37-325, $4.95, U.S.A.)
M.J. Saffon   (L37-326, $5.95, Canada)

Now you can give yourself all the beautifying effects of a face lift—safely and naturally without surgery—through a unique series of exercises created by an international beauty expert. In just minutes a day, you can smooth the forehead, banish frown lines, round out hollow cheeks, prevent puffy eyelids, erase crow's feet, remove a double chin, tighten neck muscles, and much more.

IMPROVE YOUR HEALTH
WITH WARNER BOOKS

LOW SALT SECRETS FOR
YOUR DIET
by Dr. William J. Vaughan

(L37-223, $3.95, U.S.A.)
(L37-358, $4.50, Canada)

Not just for people who must restrict salt intake, but for everyone! Forty to sixty million Americans have high blood pressure, and nearly one million Americans die of heart disease every year. Hypertension, often called the silent killer, can be controlled by restricting your intake of salt. This handy pocket-size guide can tell you at a glance how much salt is hidden in more than 2,600 brand-name and natural foods.

EARL MINDELL'S VITAMIN BIBLE
by Earl Mindell

(L30-626, $3.95, U.S.A.)
(L32-002, $4.95, Canada)

Earl Mindell, a certified nutritionist and practicing pharmacist for over fifteen years, heads his own national company specializing in vitamins. His VITAMIN BIBLE is the most comprehensive and complete book about vitamins and nutrient supplements ever written. This important book reveals how vitamin needs vary for each of us and how to determine yours; how to substitute natural substances for tranquilizers, sleeping pills, and other drugs; how the right vitamins can help your heart, retard aging, and improve your sex life.

THE CORNER DRUGSTORE
by Max Leber

large format paperback:
(L97-989, $6.95, U.S.A.)
(L37-278, $8.50, Canada)

In simple, down-to-earth language, THE CORNER DRUGSTORE provides complete coverage of the over-the-counter products and services available at your local pharmacy. Here's everything you should know about everything that pharmacies sell, a working knowledge that will save you money and enable you to use nonprescription drugs and health aids more wisely.

IMPORTANT BOOKS FOR YOUR BODY
FROM WARNER BOOKS